Therapeutic Interventions in Three Sentences

Following tenets set out by Milton Erickson, *Therapeutic Interventions in Three Sentences: Reshaping Ericksonian Hypnotherapy by Talking to the Brain and Body* presents an array of short, effective commands which have been developed for use in connection with a wide range of mental and psychosomatic disorders.

Examining in detail the basic building blocks which must be in place in order for someone to send an effective command to his or her sub-conscious mind, the book presents an elegant way of using informal variations of Ericksonian hypnotherapy in conscious states and transferring these principles to a variety of therapeutic settings. The methods described follow specific rules derived from hypnotherapy but can be integrated into any other form of counselling or therapy and can be used in short sessions, in telephone consultations and with patients in critical states, as well as conversations of a therapeutic nature by non-therapeutic professionals. The book explains why and how these interventions work, their general structure and how they can be used to tackle specific needs such as trauma, depression and anxiety disorders.

The book will be of great interest to counsellors, doctors and therapists of different orientations who are looking for therapeutic methods that can be used in short sessions or with patients in critical states, as well as non-therapeutic professionals who engage in conversations of a therapeutic nature, such as social workers, pastors, nurses, carers and teachers (including SEN teachers).

Stefan Hammel is a child and family therapist, hypnotherapist and a chaplain in a psychiatric hospital and a general hospital in Kaiserslautern, Germany. He leads seminars and workshops on therapeutic storytelling, hypnotherapy and systemic counselling around the world. For further information, please visit www.stefanhammel.com.

Therapeutic Interventions in Three Sentences

Reshaping Ericksonian Hypnotherapy by Talking to the Brain and Body

Stefan Hammel

Translated by Joanne Reynolds

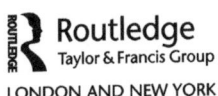

Routledge
Taylor & Francis Group

LONDON AND NEW YORK

First published in English 2020
by Routledge
2 Park Square, Milton Park, Abingdon, Oxon, OX14 4RN

and by Routledge
52 Vanderbilt Avenue, New York, NY 10017

Routledge is an imprint of the Taylor & Francis Group, an informa business

English edition © 2020 Stefan Hammel

English translation by Joanne Reynolds.

First published in German as *Grüßen Sie Ihre Seele! Therapeutische
Interventionen in drei Sätzen*

© 2017 Klett-Cotta

British Library Cataloguing-in-Publication Data
A catalogue record for this book is available from the British Library

Library of Congress Cataloging-in-Publication Data
A catalog record for this book has been requested

ISBN: 978-0-367-34202-9 (hbk)
ISBN: 978-1-003-00165-2 (ebk)

Typeset in Times New Roman
by Apex CoVantage, LLC

Contents

Introduction

Naaman, or: surely it can't be that simple!

In the days of the ancient Assyrians, a leader named General Naaman once contracted a skin disease. "He has leprosy," whispered his servants, and kept as far away from him as they possibly could. General Naaman asked his personal physician for advice, but no cure was forthcoming. The disease was starting to spread further and further over his body, and his appearance was becoming more and more disfigured. One day a maidservant mentioned that a prophet named Elisha, who was able to heal such diseases thanks to his divine powers, lived in the land of Judah, and the news was passed on to the general. He was filled with fresh hope, and set out on the road to Judah. After many days' travelling, he arrived at the prophet's house with horses and chariots and many gifts. One of the prophet's disciples came to greet them at the door and said, "My master greets you. He says that you must wash yourself seven times in the River Jordan, and your flesh will be restored and you will be cleansed." Naaman was angered by these words; "I thought that he would surely come out to me and stand and call on the name of the Lord his God, wave his hand over the spot and cure me of my leprosy. Are not the rivers of Damascus better and more splendid than this miserable stream? Could not I wash in them and be cleansed?" And he turned and made to ride away in a rage. But his servants went to him and said, "Master, if the prophet had told you to do some great thing, would you not have done it? How much more, then, when he tells you to do something so small." So the general dismounted and dipped himself in the River Jordan seven times, as the man of God had told him, and his flesh was restored and became clean like that of a young boy.[1]

Why was the general initially reluctant to go along with the treatment? If I can be forgiven for analysing this ancient story from a modern perspective, I can identify two potential reasons.

Firstly, Naaman did not feel as though the proper amount of respect had been paid, either to him or to his illness – the prophet moved straight to the solution, ignoring the visitor and his life history and suffering, and not making any effort to get to know him or listen to him. Many people resent being treated like this, even though in actual fact focusing on solutions rather than on problems often delivers a much faster outcome. When we get it the wrong way around, as sometimes happens, we can spend far too long thinking about a client's problems before we start to search together for solutions to these problems – even though the solutions were ready and waiting right from the start. In yet other cases, clients seem to regard a solution or cure as an expression of disrespect for their inner self, as though this inner self were "married" to the problem in some sense.

Secondly, the prophet offered a solution which sounded much too simple and much too illogical, and the general perceived it as an insult to his intelligence. He wanted to tackle some great feat which would test his capabilities to the limit, if not surpass them.

Sometimes it is difficult to convince people that complex problems can have simple solutions.

Note

1 Based on 2 Kings 5:9–14.

I   How to say "hello" to the mind

Regardless of whether we use the term "psyche" ("identity", "personality", "mentality") or "body" ("metabolism", "brain", "genetic material") to refer to the human organism, few would challenge the assertion that the complexity of this organism goes far beyond our powers of description. Our thinking consciousness is merely a small fragment of this whole, and one which is unable to understand the whole and intervene in it in any truly meaningful way. Given the painfully obvious limitations of our conscious mind, how then can we identify solutions for a complex organism which has been unable to identify any such solutions itself?

Any answer we find to this conundrum must be *simple* enough to do justice to the limited nature of our mind, yet *complex* enough to do justice to the complexity of the organism as a whole.

A potential answer could be to make requests of the body – asking it to distinguish between things, establish links, rearrange things, introduce regulatory mechanisms or prioritise certain things – without prescribing exactly how these requests should be performed, and without couching the requests as rigid and mandatory commands.

The imagery of dreams, and our physical and emotional experiences, might serve as an appropriate arena for an encounter between our thinking self and the remainder of our brain and body. The languages of our body, of our emotions and of our dreams might serve as a meeting place and a bridge between the deep and mysterious dimension of our body and mind and the waking consciousness of our thinking self.

It is sensible to assume that the human organism is a unit within which a *single* language is spoken, or that there are interpreters that translate messages between the organism's various subsystems in order to allow the body to function as a whole. Based on this assumption, we can expect that any suggestions made by the thinking self to the rest of the human organism will be understood by this latter, and implemented wherever possible and expedient.

The greetings in this book allow the organism itself to decide on the "how" of self-regulation and self-healing, and how (notwithstanding the limited capacities of the thinking self) it might care for itself more effectively in the future.

By leaving that which is beyond the capacities of the thinking self to the mysterious inner world of the mind and the body (sometimes referred to as the "unconscious"), the greetings in this book provide our thinking self with a tool to support the organism as a whole in its work.

Greetings as ultra-short hypnosis

Milton Erickson sometimes also used greetings of only a few sentences in length instead of the hypnosis-based treatment (or other type of treatment) which his client was expecting, and the outcomes of these interventions were very similar to those in the story about Naaman and Elisha. A woman suffering from psoriasis once came to see Erickson at his practice. Erickson examined the affected area of skin and said to her; "You've got a little psoriasis and a lot of emotions. You're alive, you've got emotions; a lot of emotions on your arms, on your body, and you've called it 'psoriasis.' So you can't have but one-third as much as you think you have." The woman was angry with Erickson for a full two weeks, until she noticed that her psoriasis had disappeared.[1]

I began many years ago to talk to the parts of my own body as a form of self-hypnotic conditioning. For example, I asked my foot – in which I was experiencing pulsating pains – "Please try greatly contracting the time during which you experience pain and greatly expanding the pain-free intervals."[2] I said to my tooth, which had become hypersensitive after treatment, "Dear molar tooth, you're right to tell me if something is troubling you, but your job is to hurt when you are injured. The sensations you're producing at the moment are inappropriate because they belong to an earlier time. Picture that dental treatment very clearly in your mind for one last time, and take the pain which you are now producing back there . . . and leave it there in that situation, which you experienced once but which is now in the past."[3] Both times the pain went away within minutes, despite having persisted for months by that point. It was also around this time that I began experimenting with the idea of encouraging sick and healthy parts of the body to talk to one another so that the sick parts could learn from the healthy what being "healthy" really meant,[4] and these interventions also proved very successful.

The first client with whom I remember using greetings was a 10-year-old girl who was so caught up in her dream world that she was absent in all but body for her schoolteachers and fellow pupils. I asked her what her brain was called, and suggested that she should ask it the following question: "Dear

Mrs Brain, could you make sure I always concentrate when my teacher is explaining the homework we need to do?" Mrs Brain would naturally answer, "Of course I can, dear Anna, you should have asked me before!" Anna would then say, "I see – but now I am asking you" and Mrs Brain would answer "Absolutely, dear Anna!"[5]

The first time that I experimented with greetings in the narrower sense of the word was when I was accompanying a client to the door of the therapy room after his therapy session had ended. This particular patient was suffering from an obsessive belief that a member of his family would fall ill with a serious disease, and that he would not notice in time to help them. While we were saying our goodbyes, I remarked casually to him, "And don't forget to pass on my greetings to your fear. I think that it has already done a great deal for you, and maybe even earned a holiday in recognition of its service. Do you think your fear would be willing to accept this expression of gratitude if you suggested the idea? It can take a mobile phone along just in case, and you can give it a call if you need any advice." When we next saw each other, the client reported the following: "I've been feeling better since our last session. Whenever I started to feel anxious, I simply thought about what you told me to say to my fear." I started to use more and more interventions of this kind with the client, and the problem resolved itself within a few sessions.[6]

As time went on, I discovered that clients implemented more or less every greeting I sent to their brain, body, mind, fears or allergies, with astonishing precision, thoroughness and permanency.[7] In most cases, the outcome of using these greetings is the same as putting the client into a deep trance and suggesting that upon waking he or she will have the behaviours and experiences referred to in the greeting and will retain them in the future.

This leads to an obvious question: what is the point of hypnosis, if the same outcome can be obtained using an alternative method in a shorter space of time? Based on observations such as those described, nowadays I rarely use traditional hypnosis techniques which involve inducing a deep trance. In no way do I wish to dispute the merit of working with hypnosis, however; instead, I regard the effectiveness of "greetings to the mind" as further evidence of its value, since they are after all a form of ultra-short hypnosis.

Setting the stage for greetings

It goes without saying that the desired outcome of interventions of this kind can only be achieved and reinforced if the stage is set and an appropriate script devised.

Let me explain using a metaphor: a film could be reduced down to one central scene, and a well-disposed audience might be willing to listen to a brief explanation of what happened before and what will happen afterwards. Yet a cinema experience of this kind would have a much less lasting impact on the audience than if the groundwork had been properly laid for this scene, and if it had in turn served as a basis for purposeful movement of the plot line towards a memorable end.

To use a different metaphor; one would not simply scatter seeds on an untilled field and then leave them to their fate without any further care or attention – and the interventions described in this book also need an appropriate environment if they are to grow and thrive. A number of ideas for increasing the metaphorical harvest of short interventions are therefore outlined here.

Most of the measures which help to make short interventions effective are themselves short interventions; the following have proven particularly useful.

1   In my experience, it is a good idea to encourage the client to adopt an attitude of anticipation paired with curiosity and suspense. For example, it is possible to:

- tell the client that significant improvements tend to take place as early as between the preliminary telephone appointment and the first session, and ask him or her to watch out for them,[8]
- refer to the fact that the process "might be surprisingly fast," or state that the effect of an intervention you intend to carry out is "likely to be quite astonishing,"
- express regret that "there's not much money to be earned from a case like yours,"
- express curiosity and joyful anticipation before and during key interventions, using facial expressions, gestures, breathing and voice,
- describe perceivable differences in the client's spontaneous behaviour, and then ask questions which convey your expectations; "I see you are now breathing much more deeply. What do you think has changed?",
- breathe out with a sigh of relief in order to encourage the client's unconscious mind to experience this sense of relief at the same time.

2   In traumatic situations, people learn new and often unhelpful patterns of behaviour in a matter of seconds; these patterns of behaviour are then retained in unchanged form for decades, even when the sufferer has long since forgotten what triggered them in the first place. Since this is the case, why should it not also be possible for alternative patterns of

behaviour – this time more helpful – to be learned within a matter of seconds and to last a lifetime? Short interventions are more effective in a therapeutic sense if they:

- can be experienced at an emotional level,
- can be perceived in sensory terms (i.e. they relate to things which can be seen, heard, touched),
- can be located in space,
- are action-focused, and
- are staged dramatically.

These elements are already clearly visible in the story of Naaman and Elisha, they are the cornerstones of many of the treatment methods used by Milton Erickson, and they can be put to a multitude of different and effective uses in a therapeutic setting.

Although it is important for therapeutic interventions of this kind to appeal to the emotions and have a dramatic staging, this does not mean that patients suffering from painful memories must undergo pain during therapy if the treatment is to be effective. It is never a good idea to force clients to revisit stressful situations or the feelings they experienced during these situations, and it is always possible to structure courses of trauma therapy in such a way that the client is protected against reliving such immense pain.

3   There is a direct relationship between the level of confidence felt by a client when he or she leaves the therapy room at the end of a session and the stability with which the effects of the therapy persist. I have therefore found it useful to address the client's "inner sceptics" in a spirit of respect and concern, using one of the following approaches:

- appointing them as "guardians who protect against disappointment," as "internal scientists," or as "quality managers,"
- distinguishing their good intentions from the paradoxical outcomes,
- dissociating them and consigning them to the past and to unreality as "what might at one point have been your inner sceptics,"
- assigning the "inner sceptics" seats in the same room but outside the client's body, as "external observers,"
- offering inner persons "who still have objections" positions as "Minister for Confidence" or "Minister of Science," and
- undermining sceptical tendencies through friendly reminders to be "sceptical about scepticism."[9]

4   We sometimes forget that clients also encounter "external sceptics"; parents, spouses, general practitioners (GPs), psychiatrists, other psychotherapists, alternative practitioners, carers, self-help groups, fortune

tellers, fellow patients and "experts" on internet forums. It is likely that clients will be faced with situations in which the people who play an important role in their lives express explicit or implicit doubts about outcomes to date, and the long-term success of therapeutic work depends on whether these doubts can be counteracted by a belief that what has already been achieved will persist and become more robust in the future. The following ideas can be helpful in this connection:

- The counsellor can say, using his or her own words, "You've experienced the effects of the therapy within your own body. It's only to be expected that your wife (or husband) will not expect it to work as quickly as you know that it can. There are many doctors and therapists who don't know that so much can be achieved so quickly. Do you think that your mind would be able to keep this in mind by saying to itself, 'They aren't in a position to understand yet. I need to be patient with them. They'll understand later'?"

- In the case of patients undergoing treatment in hospital, there can be a mutually reinforcing feedback loop between the patient's view of himself or herself and the hospital staff's view of the patient, or in other words between the verbal and non-verbal behaviour of the patient and that of the staff. The more the patient is regarded and treated as needy (ill, addicted etc.), the more he or she will behave like a needy (ill, addicted etc.) person and vice versa; in such cases it is a good idea to encourage both sides to be confident in the patient's resources. Another point worth remembering is that the opinions of the different members of staff involved also tend to undergo a process of alignment and mutual reinforcement over time. The following can be said to these members of staff (and to the patient, with the appropriate modifications): "Some of the things I observed today made me think that this patient might be ready to be discharged next week. I'm sure you'll agree with me if you take a close look yourself!" It is likely that the patient's condition will improve and that his or her stay will significantly reduce in length, in line with the prediction.

- The same approach can be adopted for out-patients, for example by telling a child undergoing treatment that you are confident that he or she will make a good and rapid recovery, and then reiterating this belief to the parents during a later telephone conversation and asking them to keep an eye on any changes.

5   Before introducing interventions aimed at bringing about change, it is often necessary to acknowledge and honour the suffering which the

client has endured as a result of the relevant situation. This does not need to involve a lengthy speech:

- "I can see how much you are suffering. If I may, I would like to suggest something to help you to feel better again . . ."
- "Many clients and even some therapists believe that the longer you have suffered, the longer the therapy needs to last; that the more complex the problem, the more involved the solution needs to be; and that the more horrible the experience you endured, the more difficult the treatment needs to be. Fortunately for us, that's not true at all. The complexity or duration of the original stressful situation has nothing to do with the complexity or duration of the therapy. Often it's the other way around – long-standing and major traumas can be resolved astonishingly quickly."
- "Perhaps an internal voice is saying to you, 'If it were really as easy as all that, I would have thought of it myself.' Perhaps the very reason you haven't been able to think of it yourself is because you have been suffering so much, and perhaps the solution ultimately appears simple, but the difficult part was finding it."
- "I hope what I'm about to say is okay with you – please tell me if otherwise. I've been wondering what your father must have suffered during his childhood in order to become the person who did something so terrible to you."

6   Before introducing novel interventions which are likely to depart from the client's expectations, it is a good idea to make it clear that you are taking both him or her and yourself seriously, and perhaps also to ask his or her permission to try something out of the ordinary:

- "I know that you were using the term 'sinking ship' in a figurative rather than a literal sense when you were talking about your life, but what do you think this ship might look like if you were to imagine it vividly in your mind's eye?"
- "I'd like to use this one particular method with you. I hope you don't take it as a sign that I've gone crazy. I'm only doing it because I know that it is more effective than certain other methods you might regard as perfectly normal. Is that okay?"
- "I'd like to tell you a story although I know you are no longer a child. This is a special story, however – one that is used in couple therapy, and one that can also be used for medical hypnosis. Can I tell it to you?"
- "I sometimes use a method based on Lego, which is extremely effective when treating children. I don't think it would really be

appropriate for you. After all, we're not children any longer – are we?"

- "I can offer you a perfectly reasonable, slow and generally ineffective method to treat your problem, or a method which is out of the ordinary, unreasonable, bizarre – and fast. Which would you prefer?"

- "I might interrupt you frequently, but that's not because I'm being rude or because I'm not interested in what you're saying – it's simply so that we can make progress as quickly as possible. Will that be OK with you?"

7   It has also proven helpful to reframe any setbacks reported by clients, putting a new and positive spin on them:

- "You said that the effects of the therapy session lasted for two days, and then things got worse again. People typically find that the effects recede a little after two or three days, but that things are still better than they were before – it evens out somewhere in the middle. Maybe we should try something today to ensure that you get to keep 80%, 90% or maybe even 95% of the effects. What do you think?"

- "When clients definitely feel worse than they did before their last session, it's generally the case that an event of some kind has occurred and caused problems; if that is true for you, it would be a good idea for us to work on it. When exactly did you start to feel worse? What happened on that day, or on the day before?"

- "During our last session we worked on the numbness, but we obviously didn't do enough about the overwhelming grief which underlies it. Now it's time for us to start working on that."

The effectiveness of greetings can therefore be heightened by ensuring that certain framework conditions are in place. As a basic principle, it is a good idea to:

- build on whatever the client is currently experiencing,
- instil positive expectations,
- promote an attitude of curiosity, searching and leaning,
- destabilise scepticism and experiences of stress and deficit,
- stabilise any emerging feelings of optimism, and
- promote any resource-focused or solution-focused experiences.

All of the interventions which follow this approach can also be framed as greetings to the unconscious mind, and multiple different greetings can be used, creating a network of helpful interventions which stabilise one another.

The structure of greetings

Greetings typically have a sender, a bearer and a recipient; a distinction can also be made between dissociative, associative and transformative greetings.

I refer to greetings as dissociative if they separate parts of a client's experience which previously tended to be viewed as linked:

> Please tell your grief that people can love and be loyal and constant without needing to feel pain or lethargy. The love they feel can exceed the pain by far, and people can live out the values they hold dearest without the kind of side effects you've been experiencing up until now.

I refer to greetings as associative if they link things together which previously tended to be viewed as separate:

> Tell your body that during each school lesson it should play imaginary football games against teams representing your boredom. One school day has six lessons, which means you'll be playing a tournament against six different teams. Whenever you wake up out of a daydream and realise that you have no idea what the teacher just said, your boredom scores a goal. Whenever you raise your hand and speak, you score a goal.

I refer to greetings as transformative if they do not link or separate parts of the client's life, but instead use something resembling an inner film to change them gradually from stressful to liberating experiences:

> Send a greeting to your self-confidence from the person hidden within you who secretly knows what you are really capable of doing: it is like a small green bud which will one day grow into a beautiful rose. What is your favourite colour?

Those who are welcomed in and those who are asked to leave

When using greetings, I often ask a client to imagine "inner persons" who can be asked to leave the client's body, or potential future versions of himself or herself who currently exist in "the world of endless opportunities" and who can be welcomed into the room and invited to merge with the client. I tailor my descriptions of these persons to the therapeutic goal and the therapeutic needs which are most pressing at that time. They might be utilised as the recipients or bearers of a greeting, or to illustrate a situation which the client is currently experiencing and to which the greeting relates.

The persons asked to leave the client's body are treated with the utmost possible respect; if it makes the client feel better, they can also remain outside his or her body on a permanent basis, since every outside is simply a different inside in the world of the mind.

The various life choices open to the client can likewise be personified, brought into the room and identified with the client's experiences, allowing the client to encounter himself or herself as the person who he or she could be, regardless of whether this person has existed in the past; if an experience of this kind proves useful from the client's perspective, it can be stabilised. The person "who you would be if all the bad things had never happened, and who you feel yourself to be when you put yourself in your own shoes" can be asked to leave "the world of possibilities and supposed impossibilities" and to enter the room, and the client can gradually familiarise himself or herself with the experiences of this person until they are ultimately perceived as the client's own.

Finally, stressful experiences which are personified and removed from the client by means of a greeting can be transformed into liberating life choices in a short mental film.[10]

The language of greetings

The language I use in this book is based on my experiences in the field of hypnotherapy.

Certain greetings rely on complex phraseology; simpler phrases would also work, but many of the added details increase the effectiveness of the greetings yet further or combine several related steps in a single one.

Participants at my seminars sometimes ask whether such complex greetings can be comprehended and implemented by clients. Based on my observations, greetings can still be implemented even if they are phrased in so complex a way that the client can no longer consciously follow what has been said. Greetings which are so complicated as to be incomprehensible induce a trance of confusion, which promotes the implementation of what has been said.[11] In my experience, it is possible and effective to use an arbitrary number of greetings and any conceivable combination of dissociative, associative and transformative greetings in juxtaposition, one after another.

The same applies when greetings are used (perhaps after seeking the client's consent) at high speed one after another, making it impossible for the client to grasp the details consciously; the messages contained in these greetings are nevertheless implemented.[12]

The preceding paragraphs approached dissociative and associative greetings primarily from the perspective of verbal language; I would now like to discuss in more detail a number of principles of linguistic usage which apply when developing dissociative and associative greetings.

Separating problems, connecting solutions

The main rule I follow when developing greetings can be summarised as "separate problems, connect solutions."

"Separating problems" can entail any of the following:

1   dividing something which appears to be a *single* problem into its component parts,
2   creating a stronger distinction between problems which have already been identified as separate,
3   separating problems from concepts of self, of the felt reality, of the here and the now, and describing them in terms of "someone you can be," "something that could be," "over there" and "back then,"
4   distinguishing problems from resources, and stressful aspects of a problem from potentially helpful ones.

"Connecting solutions" can entail any of the following:

1   reinforcing solution-focused and resource-focused experiences, and emphasising them as important, profound, current, plausible and relevant,
2   linking several resources associatively,
3   identifying resources with the current experience of self and reality,
4   linking reinforced resources with the experience of fragmented problems.

Signal words can be used to separate terms which are closely associated with the problem in question on the one hand, and the experience of self on the other; instead of referring to "pain," reference can be made to "potential pain" or "previous pain," for example.

Similarly, terms which are associated with the desired solution-focused experience can be linked to the experience of self. Instead of talking about "your pain," the therapist can use the phrase "your desire for relief and improved well-being."

Similarly, the component parts of a solution can be associated and the component parts of a problem dissociated by using:

•   grammatical constructions such as modal and non-modal verbs,
•   adverbs relating to place, time and manner,

- past, present or future tense, and the first, second or third person,
- indirect speech and techniques of concretion and abstraction.

Signal words can also be used to separate parts of the problem as it is experienced by the client from each other and from the experience of self. Dissociation can be achieved:

1   through use of the third person ("someone", "your body", "part of you"),
2   spatially, using terms such as "over there", "somewhere", "outside you",
3   chronologically, using terms such as "previously", "it was", "in 100 years",
4   by shifting from reality into unreality ("would be", "hypothetical", "theoretical", "assuming that"),
5   by moving to another level of reality ("you say that . . .", "people say that . . ."),
6   through abstraction, using terms such as "these symptoms", "these phenomena",
7   by referring to the opposite, using terms such as "not good", "very unpleasant", "discomfort".

Conversely, signal words can be used to link together the component parts of a solution-focused experience with each other and with the experience of self. Association can be achieved:

1   through use of the second person ("you"),
2   spatially, using terms such as "here", "in you", "in your place",
3   chronologically, using terms such as "now", "from now on", "forever", "eternally true",
4   by emphasising the reality of the situation ("is", "really", "actually", "remarkably"),
5   by focusing on original experiences ("you feel", "you perceive"),
6   through concretion, using terms such as "this particular", "precisely this",
7   by using positive phrases ("pleasant", "enjoy", "trust").

Very different effects can be achieved by using the second person or the third person.

Firstly, problems are experienced less intensely when they are described in the third person ("Your body is in pain") than when they are described in the second person ("You are in pain").

Secondly, use of the second person tends to mean that the message is received by the conscious mind with its limited possibilities, while use of the third person means that the unconscious mind – with its significantly greater potential for creating change – feels called upon. Clients therefore tend to protest and discuss endless details if we voice suggestions in the second person, whereas this tends not to be the case with suggestions in the third person. For example, a client would probably protest if a therapist said, "Maybe if you tried to feel less pain and more comfort?" He or she might have more faith in the process if the therapist said, "Maybe if you ask your body to create less pain and more comfort, do you think it might be willing to do that for you?" In my experience, suggestions formulated in the third person are implemented more frequently and more consistently by the body.

The third person can therefore also be used to introduce potentially helpful ideas while circumventing objections which might otherwise nip fresh hope or a new learning experience in the bud before it has had the opportunity to blossom. "Please send a greeting to your arm, and suggest that it might try spreading its good sensations to the back, which hasn't been doing so well lately." Once the positive experience has been established in this way, we can naturally reinforce it by returning to the second person: "How about if your back imagines experiencing this good feeling, just as though it has felt this way for months, and how about if you listen to your back – has anything changed?"

Similarly, we can respond to scepticism by allowing the client to experience the good things about a fictitious future or a secondary level of reality, and then switching to the present and what is currently being experienced: "Imagine that in some distant or near future your back is feeling better. How do you hold your body? What do you look like? What kind of things do you do more often than before?"

Modal and non-modal verbs can be used in an analogous way. If we want to invite a client to anticipate new opportunities, to test them out and to examine their effects, we can use modal verbs to introduce these ideas ("assuming that it might be so . . .", "in theory it could be the case that . . .") and then – as soon as the sentence has slipped past the client's sceptical bodyguard as an apparently fictitious assumption – moving to non-modal verbs: "And when you imagine that, how does it feel? While you feel like that, what can you do now that was perhaps impossible before?"

The use of metaphors and idioms

The bodyguard metaphor I used in the previous paragraph illustrates the way that processes such as those explained previously can also be represented using metaphors, parables and illustrative examples from nature, technology and the whole panoply of human life. The bodyguard can of course be addressed in person, and greetings sent to him or her:

> Let's imagine that there is a bodyguard watching over you, one who doesn't want you to be disappointed – he's certainly doing a very thorough job, isn't he! Could you ask him to do one extra task by making sure that he does not accidentally create disappointment by warning you about the potential for disappointment when things might otherwise have turned out well – would he be able to stop doing that?

The bodyguard metaphor would then serve as a role model for various processes within the body. Functional models can also be used in a similar way:

> The difference between what is and what would be is not as clear as you might think. Everything is and everything would be, and everyone has a different take on it. "Is" and "would be" are like two different compartments in your brain. It might be a good idea to move some of the unhelpful attitudes, expectations and interpretations of life which were previously in the "is" compartment into the "would be" compartment, and to move some of the positive expectations and interpretations which were previously in the "would be" compartment into the "is" compartment. Your conscious mind might not be able to do that, but your unconscious mind will know how. Send a greeting to your brain, and say that it should start preparing for this new sorting procedure. We'll come back to it later – for the time being there's something else we need to discuss. . .

What was achieved using signal words, grammatical constructions and two different metaphorical models can also be achieved using the voice, the manner of speaking and body language as a whole.

The use of non-verbal communication

Body language, the voice and the manner of speaking can have an enormous impact on the meaning expressed by a greeting. For example, the therapist can heighten the effect of a greeting by moving his or her hands as though he or she were taking things apart, putting them together, making them smaller or larger or otherwise reshaping them.

He or she might say,

> Send the following message to your grieving mind: you feel and you can continue to feel this much love and loyalty [using our hands to indicate a large amount, and gesturing towards the right-hand side of the body], but your mind can regulate the pain independently [moving

our gaze to the left, and using our hands on the left-hand side to indicate a smaller amount], and it can be smaller than the love and loyalty [suddenly moving our gaze to the right, and once again using our hands on the right-hand side to indicate a larger amount].

Movements of the hands can be used to show how parts of the client's experience can be shaped, reproduced, moved to other areas, collected from different areas and brought together in a single location. Stressful experiences can be placed in boxes or drawers, which can be closed (carefully or with reckless abandon) so that the contents are stored safely and can be moved to a different location later if necessary.

If you wish to convey these processes using head, hand and eye movements while working with a client, it is a good idea to shift attention on a regular basis from the content of what you are saying to your gestures and facial expressions while you are saying it.

The voice can also be used to foster positive expectations. A quiet, low voice can be used during the first part of a sentence, while casually referring to the client's previous symptoms, and then a powerful, confident voice during the second part of the sentence, while explaining that none of us have ever visited the future. This technique of using two different manners of speaking allows us to differentiate between the certainty of the memory and the alleged certainty of the expectation, and opens up the idea that the future might be better than expected – and this potentially good future is also given precedence over the unpleasant memory through the way that the voice is used. All of this happens without needing to discuss every last detail of the processes in question with the client, since for the most part they take place in the client's unconscious mind.[13]

The sender of the greeting

The sender of a greeting is generally the therapist: "Send a greeting to your left hand."

Variations on this theme are naturally also possible:

My cat wishes to send a friendly greeting to your cells, and to say that what's been happening has nothing to do with her. What you thought was a cat hair allergy was simply a misunderstanding on the part of your body. . .

Or:

Your right hand could send a greeting to your left hand, and say that it would like to take lessons from it and learn how it moves its thumb so elegantly. Do you think your right hand would be happy to send your left hand a greeting of this kind?

A greeting of this kind involves multiple dissociations, meaning that the client's conscious mind is circumvented – together with any objections it might raise as to whether the left hand can really learn from the right hand how to move its thumb. Given that these objections are often the only barrier to success, this can be a very useful strategy.[14]

The bearer of the greeting

The client is generally the conveyor of a greeting which the therapist asks to be passed on to an inner something or someone: "Send a greeting to your mind."

Of course, we could also say: "Dear right hand, please could you tell the left hand . . ."

By referring to parts of the body (such as the hand) as subjects using the second person when we would normally refer to them as objects using the third person, we can dissociate the hand from the client's experience of self. This partially removes the hand from the control of the conscious mind with its limited possibilities, and allows it to act as a representative of the unconscious mind with its unlimited possibilities.

It is also possible to ask the person "who you are now while you are feeling well in yourself" to take a message to the person "who you were back then" or "who you will be in a while."

Finally, it is also possible to use an angel or a loved one who has passed away as a bearer of greetings: "I will send along an angel who will comfort you when . . ."[15] The therapist can decide whether to frame this as a thought exercise or as a spiritual practice, depending on his or her own beliefs and (more importantly) those of the client.

The recipient of the greeting

Greetings are always addressed to recipients in the third person. If I address a client as "you," he or she will tend to respond on the level of conscious thought and experience. If I distinguish entities such as "your brain," "your mind" and "your immune system" from this "you," parts of his or her involuntary and unconscious experience will tend to respond, providing access to many different routes of action which are not available to us on a conscious level.

Instead of parts of the body (in the broader sense of the term) such as "mind," "fear," "lungs" or "brain," imaginary persons can also be invented;

the outcome of doing so appears to be that the body then discovers them or spontaneously creates them. In the section on food, addiction and habits, for example, a greeting is sent to the person who "knows what a healthy weight looks like."

Clients can be asked, "Send a message to your deceased mother in your thoughts . . .", "Send a message to your grandfather in the world beyond this one, and ask him to do you a favour . . ." or (if the recipient has not yet left this world) "Send a greeting to the image of your father in your head, or what we could call the father within you . . ."

Greetings addressed to bacteria can be used to strengthen the immune system by announcing that a counter-attack is imminent, or by dismissing them from their work and sending them on holiday – somewhere outside the body. Even if the bacteria do not hear the greeting, the immune system will follow the instructions embodied within it.

When metaphors or parables are used, greetings can be sent to a metaphorical character – and the body will find or create an inner person who corresponds to this character. The section on the muscular system contains the following greeting:

> After a sailing ship has weathered a storm, it sails into a dock so that all the rigging can be tuned up. The cordage is loosened and tightened and then loosened again and tightened again, over and over again until everything is just right. Please tell the workers that they're doing a great job!

Representatives of the client's unconscious mind are addressed as dock workers in this instance, but the client's own metaphors can also be used; if a client refers to himself or herself as a "scaredy-cat," a greeting could be sent both to the "scaredy-cat" and the "big bold cat," for example, and if a client refers to himself or herself as a "wallflower," a greeting could be sent to the "exquisite bloom which radiates a beauty that is true, deep and whole."

People often ask me whether it makes a difference if greetings are addressed to "the brain," "the mind," "the inner world" or "the unconscious." There can be little doubt that a greeting addressed to "the leg" will have a different effect to one addressed to "your grief"; a different authority within the body will respond and react in each case. As yet, however, I have not identified any major differences in the effect of very broad terms such as "the brain" and "the mind." Nevertheless, I always take the client's individual preferences into account when selecting the recipient of a greeting; I will address "the soul" when working with more spiritually minded clients, "the mind" or "the brain" when working with people who have a scientific bent, and "the unconscious" when working with people who have come to me looking for a hypnosis practitioner.

Use of the definite article ("the") tends to have a more strongly dissociative effect than use of the possessive pronoun ("your"), which can be useful in certain circumstances; on the other hand, the possessive pronoun heightens the sense of personal relevance and the feeling that the therapist has connected with the client's concerns. Addressing a greeting to "the tinnitus" makes a greater distinction between the client and his or her symptoms than addressing a greeting to "your tinnitus." This encourages the client to make this distinction too, and may foster the internal expectation that a life is possible in which he or she does not suffer from the symptoms.

In many cases, the recipient of a greeting is also selected on the basis of the client's concerns and the therapeutic goal.

If the goal of a particular course of therapy were to reduce pain, I would tend to select the body as a whole or the affected body part as the recipient of the greeting, in order to emphasise the difference between the body or its parts and the scepticism which the client (or rather the client's experience of self) may be experiencing. My aim would be to separate out the suggestive messages being sent by these sceptical inner persons from the remaining communication happening in and with the body, and at the same time to stimulate the different persons within the body to take action independently of these sceptics.

If the goal of therapy were to tackle a problematic sleep behaviour, for example sleep apnoea, I might address a greeting to the client's sleeping self in order to activate inner persons who will become active when the client is asleep, despite the fact that they are all but unknown to the client's waking conscious.

If I were working with a client suffering from psychosis, I would address the greeting to his or her dream self in order to be sure that the impulse to change will take effect in areas which are largely separate from the non-psychotic experience (of both the client and the population in general). I might also ask him or her to send messages backwards and forwards between the dream self and the inner person who is familiar with the reality which we all share.

Identifying the response to greetings

A greeting can often be followed with a question such as "Do you think your brain will be happy with that?" or "Does your mind agree?" Clients rarely answer "no," but if they do then it provides the therapist with a valuable indication that the ideas expressed in the greeting do not fit with the client's values and desires (or the values and desires of the inner person to whom the greeting was addressed). I believe it is also useful to issue frequent reminders to the client (and to oneself) that the client is in charge, or in other words that the therapy should be adapted to meet his or her needs rather than the other way around.

Clients sometimes reply something along the lines of, "Oh, if only it were so simple . . ." When this happens, it is possible for the therapist firstly to work with the client's scepticism (see the sections on therapeutic effect and depression for greetings that can be sent to the client's inner sceptics), and then to return to the previous greeting again – with the likely outcome that the client will answer, "Yes, my brain is happy with that" or the equivalent.

Testing the effect of greetings

It is often useful to test the effect of greetings immediately, using a simple before-and-after test and observing the client's physical reactions:

Observation beforehand:

"Apologies for interrupting. I noticed that your voice suddenly faltered when you spoke about your father, and again when you spoke about the violence you experienced in your childhood. Your voice became quiet, as though it were being smothered. Could I possibly ask you to do something?"

Greeting:

"Please tell your brain that it is capable of staying surprisingly calm while remembering things that would probably have been very painful before. Do you think your brain will be OK with that?"

Test question:

"What did you want to tell me about your father and about the violence you experienced in your childhood?"

Observation afterwards:

"Apologies for interrupting again. I noticed that this time you spoke more articulately – your voice sounded clear and strong, your body was in a more upright position, you held your gaze high and looked at me with more confidence than when you talked about these matters before, and you also talked in much more detail. It's quite remarkable. I believe that your brain has immediately acted upon the greeting you sent to it. Have you noticed any changes yourself?"

When integrated into the therapeutic conversation, tests such as these heighten the effectiveness of greetings, as well as improving the quality of the therapeutic work, alerting the therapist and client to the importance of non-verbal behaviour (both that which can be seen and that which can be heard) and teaching the therapist how to gauge accurately which greetings are likely to work well with particular clients, and which are suitable for use with multiple clients.

Greetings to improve therapeutic effect

There is a direct relationship between a client's confidence in the effectiveness of therapy at the end of a session and his or her willingness to take a playful approach to doubts and not be overcome by them on the one hand, and the actual effectiveness of therapy in the long run on the other. This section contains multiple interventions aimed at fostering this confidence and willingness, and the section on depression also contains interventions which can be used to tackle scepticism.

The period between one therapy session and the next can of course sometimes throw up surprises; if a client states that "everything has stayed the same," or "things have got even worse than they were before," the suggestion implicit in these statements (i.e. that the therapeutic work carried out during the previous session was ineffective) poses a potential risk to the success of therapy. In my experience, it is always possible to find a more helpful explanation than the conclusion that "something must have gone wrong" with the therapy. A thorough investigation of the phenomenon reveals several possibilities:

1   Despite the critical statements which have been made, the client's voice and body language are more animated than before. He or she seems to be more relaxed and cheerful than during the previous session, and talks about different topics. The issues worked on last time have been resolved, but the client has become accustomed to looking for problems, and has turned to less urgent matters without consciously noticing that the more urgent ones discussed during the last session are no longer relevant.

2   The client appears to be sad, perhaps because he or she was previously in a state of numbness which has now given way to an experience of grief. The therapist can suggest to the client that grief represents progress when compared to the previous state of numbness, and discuss

with the client what he or she is grieving for and how best this grief can be handled.

3   Something has happened since the last session which means that the client is now faced with yet greater challenges. For example, if the client has "fallen off the wagon" by starting to smoke again, he or she may have suffered a bereavement since the last session and be processing the associated grief. In such cases care should be taken to avoid attributing the client's decision to start smoking again to a lack of therapeutic effect, and instead to suggest "adapting the therapeutic method slightly to ensure that you will be equipped if anything like this should ever happen again in the future."

4   The client may not have anticipated that life would continue to be a series of ups and downs. The best approach in such cases is to remind the client to compare Saturdays with Saturdays, evenings with evenings and Decembers with Decembers; for example, if he or she complains of low mood, it might be because his or her child died around this time many years ago, and the season has been a trigger for depressive feelings ever since. The client should be encouraged to focus on improvements in comparison to last year (or in comparison to last weekend, in comparison to similarly cold days last December etc.) rather than improvements since the last therapy session.

5   If none of these apply, I interpret reports of a deterioration in the client's condition as a valuable indication that there are other – hitherto unknown – issues which need to be incorporated into the therapeutic process, and I work with the client to identify any new problems which need to be worked on before the therapeutic goal can be achieved.

Providing a brief summary of the procedure and also using "greetings to the mind" can encourage the client to reinterpret the situation and redirect his or her thinking as outlined in the five cases illustrated.

Something which every therapist should remember, regardless of the style of therapy they practice, is that a client's experiences between the end of one session and the start of the next, and how he or she interprets these experiences, depend to a large extent on the expectations he or she holds regarding this period of time. Expectations typically have their basis in memories. The client's expectations regarding the period following the therapy session can be generated either from memories of the therapy session itself, or from memories of the time before the session. Clients often report that the effects of a therapy session lasted for three days or so and then disappeared, but if we follow up on statements of this kind with further questions, we learn that the effects did not in fact vanish completely after just a few days; instead, the client's condition settled down somewhere in between the low point experienced before the therapy session, and the high point experienced just after.

In order to encourage clients to generate expectations on the basis of memories, we can focus their attention on experiences which recurred over a long period of time, experiences which were particularly intense or experiences which were recent and therefore appear relevant. Paradigmatically speaking, it appears that memories which are marked in the brain as "strong" (emotionally intense), "long" (experienced for a sustained period or frequently) or "new" are particularly likely to generate expectations. It may be that therapeutic effect tends to recede after a few days because clients initially generate expectations from their memories of the recently ended therapy session, then – once these memories have faded – increasingly base their expectations on experiences which recurred many times (or which were particularly intense at one point in the distant past). As the memory of good experiences in the "new" category fades, the influence of bad memories in the "long-lasting" and "intense" categories increases in direct proportion, and the balance of expectation-generating sources shifts away from the positive new experiences. In order to increase the likelihood that these positive new memories will generate expectations and decrease the likelihood that expectations will be generated on the basis of negative old memories, I sometimes discuss this with the client; if necessary, I might also discuss which of these phenomena might have led to the apparent fall-off in therapeutic effect.

Based on my observations, the overall duration of a course of therapy and the lasting nature of its outcomes depend to a great degree on the extent to which far-reaching changes can be achieved in the first session. The client's memories of the effectiveness of this first session determine his or her expectations of how effective the following sessions will be, and these expectations are the primary determinant of what the client can actually achieve during his or her work with the therapist. It is for this reason that I advise against spending the whole of the first session asking questions about the client's past history unless they are directly related to therapeutic interventions; there are various options available for reducing the amount of time spent on such questions and increasing the amount of time spent on processes which bring about change.

All of the therapist's questions about the client's previous history and his or her responses to the client's answers can be linked consistently with interpretations and information which are designed to bring about change. Greetings are an ideal vehicle for doing so, since they only involve interrupting the work briefly.

Since neutrality is in any case impossible to achieve when requesting information, it is a good idea to use suggestive techniques to phrase client history questions in order to ensure firstly that the client's original painful experiences are given their due, and secondly that his or her attention is then shifted consistently to resources and experiences likely to generate curiosity and positive expectations. Greeting-style interventions force the unconscious mind to play a greater role than the conscious mind during this processing of gathering information, and this is particularly true when they are addressed to third-person recipients:

> "Imagine that I asked your daughter what she needed from you – what do you think she would say?"
>
> "What do you think your healthy ear would say if we asked how it does such a good job of hearing things?"
>
> "If your mind was a villa which needed to be renovated, and if you carried out an inspection of this villa with a renovation expert, which jobs would need to be carried out first, and which later? What order should they be carried out in?"

Going into detail takes time. In order to avoid wasting too much time on details of the client's past history during the early stages of therapy, he or she (or his or her unconscious mind) can be asked from time to time to adapt what is being discussed – using non-verbal resources which are unavailable to the therapist – in such a way that it better fits his or her circumstances and needs.

Using greetings on oneself

It is of course also possible to send greetings to one's own mind. In order to help the mind to distinguish them from simple thought exercises and allow particular suggestions to be implemented, it is a good idea to mark the difference between the two, for example by prefacing greetings to our own inner self with words such as "dear mind" or "dear immune system," by saying the greeting out loud, or by pausing in one's thoughts for a while to heighten the importance of the greeting by allowing it extra time.

Phrases such as "Send a greeting to your mind, and tell it . . ." can be replaced with wordings such as "Dear mind, please put these worries in the drawer of the bedside table until I have more information," or "Hello headache, please go into the big toe on my right foot and wait for me there." All of the greetings in this book can be rephrased in this way.

People sometimes claim that it is impossible to practice therapeutic methods on oneself. In my opinion, it would be closer to the truth to say that it is impossible for the conscious and thinking self to practice therapeutic methods on the remainder of the body. When working with greetings, the therapeutic challenge is delegated from the conscious (but overloaded) inner persons to unconscious (but capable) inner persons; whether or not this can serve as a replacement for therapy in individual cases is a question which does not need to be answered at this point. Suffice it to say that self-therapeutic interventions in the form of greetings are astonishingly effective.

When the mind sends back greetings

Can a simple "greeting to the mind" really achieve such astonishing effects – for example, by prompting an enuretic 11-year-old child to become dry at night from one day to the next, for the very first time in her life? If it were really so simple, would it not have been obvious to everyone from the start?

I suggest that anyone wishing to experiment with "greetings to the mind" should keep a careful record of the greetings they have used, and observe the response to these greetings very closely – in the following seconds, minutes, days and weeks.

When we send a message to ourselves or others and lay emphasis on this message, what kind of effect does it have on what we or they then do, or how we or they then feel? In my experience, few people bother to observe, compare and evaluate the effects of communication and self-communication with the consistency required to obtain definitive answers to this question.

If we observe and describe – with absolute precision – the changes which our messages bring about in the experiences of the people we encounter, and how they express these changes (in body language, behaviour and verbal feedback), it turns out that every message which is received has an effect.

In order to achieve a change of this kind, which is life-enhancing in nature, it is necessary to silence the internal and external sceptical voices whose combined effect is generally to make clients expect what they remember, and therefore end up once more with what they have already tolerated in the past.

When the mind sends greetings back, it typically does so inconspicuously – for example, by reducing the frequency of symptoms. The change will only be noticed by someone who is keeping close track of such matters, but it will then be involuntarily stabilised as a result of this careful attention.

The mind might send a greeting back by ensuring that the symptoms are triggered by higher levels of stress than was previously the case, and it will only be possible to observe such a change by comparing Mondays with Mondays and evenings with evenings, i.e. by observing whether the symptom would previously have occurred with this intensity under these conditions.

Sometimes a client will say, "The symptoms are still there," but on closer questioning respond, "Not the headache part of the migraine, just a kind of pressure behind the eyes," or "Most of the time it's not the high beeping tone, it's a sort of buzzing."

We may notice that the mind has sent a greeting back when the client tells us, "Everything is just as bad as it was before!" but then proceeds to talk to us about problems which are different to those which they complained of previously, and which appear to be less serious.

We may notice that the mind has sent a greeting back when the client tells us, "I'm really not doing well at all," but looks very different to the way he or she looked last time – with a relaxed appearance, a strong voice, an upright gait and a straight gaze.

We may notice that the mind has sent a greeting back if the client's symptoms undergo a transformation – for example, a state of numbness may be replaced by a state of grief. The client might say that he or she is feeling "particularly bad," but this shift is the first step on the path towards recovery.

Notes

1 Rosen 1982, 154–155. Distraction was one of Erickson's preferred methods. When working with patients suffering from acne, for example, he asked them to remove mirrors from their environment; when working with patients suffering from warts, he advised them to soak the relevant area in alternating hot and cold baths and later to forget the treatment and the warts. Ibid., 87–88.
2 Cf. Hammel 2019a, 60.
3 Ibid., 78. For further details regarding the use of metal placebos, cf. 35, 43–44, 47.
4 Rosemarie Dypka from Hamburg gave me some very useful pointers in this direction. Cf. Hammel 2011, 62–63, et passim.
5 Hammel 2019a, 133–134.
6 Hammel 2011, 135–136.
7 A number of these greetings, as well as observations concerning their therapeutic use, can be found in Hammel 2014, 289–292.
8 Prior 2007, 82–96.
9 Further options for identifying and using the client's sceptical thoughts in a spirit of respect can be found in Meiss 2016, 173–175.
10 This method of working with personified life choices is described in detail in Hammel 2019b.
11 Cf. for example the explanation of therapeutic double binds in Hammel 2011, 218–223.
12 The greeting "The before-and-after test" from the section on trauma can be used to check whether greetings have been implemented.
13 Commented examples of similar uses of body language, voice and manner of speaking can be found in Hammel 2014, 197–210, 245–254 and on the DVD (Hammel 2019c).
14 Hammel 2019a, 62.
15 Cf. the greeting "Heavenly homework helper" in the section on couples and family therapy, and the parting phrase "I'm sending an angel with you on your way" in Hammel 2012, 20.

II When to say "hello" to the mind

Greetings can be used to achieve significant progress towards all of the goals which clients typically wish to achieve in therapy, including those which they only reveal upon further questioning since they do not initially regard them as achievable.

Greetings can accordingly be used to heal physical or mental ailments; resolve interpersonal problems; improve attitudes to restrictions such as ageing, mortality, an uncertain future or doubts regarding a current relationship and reduce or overcome any obstacles which might stand in the way of successful therapy.

In order to allow readers of this book to identify greetings which are relevant to their work more easily, each greeting is preceded by a number of entries labelled with the abbreviations "T," "R" and "M." "T" stands for the **topics** which (in my opinion) are most pertinent to the particular greeting, e.g. "depression" or "addiction"; "R" refers to the **recipients** of a greeting, e.g. "the mind" or "the brain"; and "M" stands for the **message** conveyed by the greeting (in summary form).

Effectiveness of therapy

The purpose of the greetings in this section is to increase the effectiveness of therapeutic work, i.e. to destabilise attitudes and beliefs which prevent clients reaching their therapeutic goals, to ensure that they are not "overloaded" either during or after the therapy session and to stabilise and build upon what has already been achieved.

The amount of time available for therapeutic work is always limited, and so it is a good idea to avoid wasting this time on therapist/client question-and-answer sessions; instead, the therapist can offer vague interpretations or several different interpretations of a particular set of circumstances, and invite the client – silently, in his or her own mind – to adapt what has been said so that it better fits his or her view of the world and his or her memories, goals and desires. An invitation of this kind is formulated in the intervention "Adapt everything to make it even better."

The greeting "Only 90%" offers another option for maximising therapeutic effect; the therapist explains to the client that regardless of what is achieved during the therapy session, a certain fraction of it will probably be lost afterwards. Clients who have this explained to them tend to lose less of what has been achieved than those who are confronted with the phenomenon without having received any such prior explanation. In order to avoid causing loss through a suggestive effect, it is also possible to tell the client that although some people experience a small loss, others find that the benefits of therapy keep on growing due to spontaneous training effects, and to ask the client to identify the group into which he or she falls.

The section on depression contains additional greetings which promote positive ways of handling sceptical voices.

Adapt everything to make it even better

T: **Ethics, safety of therapy, values, effectiveness of therapy**
R: **The unconscious**
M: **You have the power within you to adjust my message in such a way that anything which does not fit your needs can still be received in the most appropriate form.**

> Tell your unconscious that it can adjust everything I say to make it a better fit for your own personal situation, even if the words I use are not entirely right.

This greeting is suitable for universal use.

Sit back and let the problem be solved

T: **Autism, effectiveness of therapy, giftedness, perfectionism, stuttering, tics, compulsive behaviour (OCD)**
R: **The mind, body, spirit (two-level greeting)**
M: **Your thinking mind cannot, but other parts of you can.**

> Greet your thinking self in a friendly manner, and tell it that it cannot solve this problem itself, but it can also invite your body and mind to take over, and simply sit back and look on with amazement as they get on with the job.

The greeting is particularly suitable for people with a strong need to stay in control, and more generally as a way of reinforcing suggestive messages. The skills needed to solve a particular problem will be searched for in parts of the body where resources are potentially available, and a distinction (i.e. separation) will be made between parts of the body which might be sceptical about any such solution and therefore unhelpful, and those which believe that solutions are possible.

Only 90%

T: **Effectiveness of therapy**
R: **The mind**
M: **A little is lost, but most is retained. What is retained grows from hour to hour.**

Greet your mind and tell it that sometimes a therapy session goes particularly well and you go home feeling really happy, but afterwards what you have achieved is partially lost, and perhaps only 80%, 90% or 95% is retained. Tell your mind that this is sometimes unavoidable, but that therapy also has a "training effect"; experience shows that more of what has been achieved in a therapy session becomes permanently available as every hour passes.

When choosing between three quantified options which appear to be of the same value, people generally choose the middle of the three. By asserting that some of the good effects of the therapy session will be lost, the therapist saves the client's inner sceptic from the trouble of coming to the same conclusion. Such an assertion sounds plausible, and helps the client to accept what is also implied, namely that most of the effects of the therapy session will be retained. The client will be so busy considering whether 80%, 90% or 95% of the effects will be retained that he or she will not question whether the percentage will indeed be this high, and his or her expectations will be adjusted accordingly. The greeting therefore reduces to around 10% the likely loss of positive expectations, which give rise to positive experiences, which give rise to positive memories, which give rise to positive expectations, and so on.

Turning the sceptic into a silent observer

T: **Scepticism, disappointment (and the desire to avoid it)**
R: **A guardian who raises objections in order to protect against disappointment**

M: **Instead of raising objections out of a desire to prevent disappointment and thereby giving rise to the very disappointment it wishes to avoid, an inner authority should observe the client silently for a period of time in a spirit of trust.**

Sometimes when people return home after a therapy session, they notice that some of the positive effects of the session have vanished. Perhaps there is part of you that wants to enjoy what you have achieved, while there is another part of you that wants to criticise and object in order to avoid being disappointed – but these criticisms and objections end up causing the very disappointment they were intended to prevent. Please tell this guardian inside you that he or she would be able to protect you against disappointment much more effectively by remaining silent for a whole week, and observing how well you get on with your life while he or she simply sits and watches.

The purpose of the greeting is to make the client more confident that the course of therapy will have the desired effects, and to invite him or her to adopt a playful attitude to any lingering doubts.

The Minister for Confidence

T: **Scepticism, disappointment (and the desire to avoid it)**
R: **The inner sceptic**
M: **You are more likely to avoid disappointment if you trust in the process than if you raise objections.**

I have the feeling that there is someone inside you who is still unsure about how much you have achieved, and how long these achievements will last. Let's imagine that this person who has been sceptical up until now leaves your body invisibly, and goes over there – now that you can see him properly, he does not seem very happy at all. If we were to ask him, "Would you like to take on the role of Minister for Confidence in Mr M.'s life?", what do you think he would say? Would he accept the appointment?

When offers of this kind are extended to inner persons, they are accepted almost without exception; the outcome is typically the disappearance of more or less all the objections that were unintentionally hampering the progress of therapy.

I belong to you and I do things differently!

T: **Borderline (BPD), family, identity, migration, trauma, compulsive behaviour (OCD)**

R: **Parents (family)**

M: **I choose both: I belong to you, and I do things differently to you!**

Send a greeting to the image of your parents which exists in your imagination, and tell them, "I choose both: I belong to you, and at the same time I do things differently than you!"

Some of the most intimidating inner sceptics are or were sceptics in the external world, including the members of a client's family of origin and their beliefs. This greeting can be varied in many different ways; it can be used to teach clients who have experienced family-related trauma to differentiate the different components of their sense of belonging to this family – for example, by amending the first part of the greeting as follows: "I belong to you in my own way," or "I belong to you in some ways." The second part of the greeting can also be adapted: ". . . and at the same time I do things differently than the way that you think they ought to be done," or ". . . than you would do them." Depending on the circumstances, the greeting can be sent to individuals, such as a parent, or to the whole family – or to the child who the client used to be. The greeting is also suitable for clients trapped in a conflict of loyalties between two different families or cultures – for example, those raised in a traditional Eastern culture who would like to adopt a more liberal and Western way of life.

Send your clone ahead

T: **Relapse prevention, stabilisation, anchor (preconscious)**

R: **The person who you want to be**

M: **The inner you is capable of recreating exactly how happy you feel now whenever you need to feel happy again, and even before you notice that you need it.**

While you're feeling happy and relaxed, imagine that a perfect copy of you – a clone – leaves your body. It goes on ahead of you into your future, and from time to time it meets the person that you will become. At the first indication that you're not feeling as happy and relaxed as you do now, the clone comes to find the person you become in the future, and fills you up with exactly the same happy feelings that you are experiencing now – regardless of whether you are asleep or awake, and without you even noticing that your happiness may have started to fade. Is it okay that the clone does that for you?

It appears to be the case that clients follow the instruction to fill themselves up with the happy feelings they are currently experiencing at the first indications of their previous troubles, since problems which are worked on in this way are rarely raised again in subsequent sessions. This may well be attributable to the greeting; since the problem has been solved at a pre-conscious level, the client remembers neither the problem nor the solution. As a general rule, greetings with a similar structure that prompt a helpful response at the first indications of disordered sleep behaviours (nightmares, night-time waking caused by depression, sleep apnoea, bedwetting), i.e. once again at an unconscious level and at the first signs of stress, are also implemented rapidly and effectively by clients.

Trauma

Trauma can arise when a person feels helplessly exposed to an existential threat at an emotional or physical level, and is so overcome by fear (or disgust) that a state of numbness ensues. It can also arise when a person observes and identifies with another person or living creature experiencing a situation of this kind.

Threats of this kind often relate to the loss of loved ones or of the sense of belonging among these loved ones, the loss of a system (such as a homeland) which has served as a source of identity or the sudden questioning of values which had previously appeared inviolate.

The sense of numbness or dissociation which accompanies a traumatic experience extends to physical movements as well as to sensations, emotions, thoughts, inner films and the sense of space and time. When remembering their past experiences, trauma sufferers generally return to the physical and mental state they were in during those experiences.

Revisiting traumatic memories during a therapy session therefore tends to place clients in the state of numbness they experienced at the time of the trauma, or an underlying state such as panic, despair or a willingness to attack. As well as being extremely stressful, states of this kind are wholly unconducive to creativity, and are therefore not suitable as a basis for therapeutic work.

There are a number of options for ensuring that clients do not return to the state they experienced during the original trauma when the topic is touched upon during a therapy session:

It is possible to work "one-step removed"[1], i.e. next to the problem situation addressed by the client, by using metaphors, or by discussing traumatic structures and potential solutions in abstract terms and linking them with proposals for resolving the trauma, taking care to avoid reactivating specific memories in the client.

It is possible to disassociate the client who experienced the trauma and work with this (imaginary) externalised and traumatised client as a figure who exists outside the client who is physically present.

It is also possible to work directly with the traumatic memories. Before doing so, it is important to suggest to the client that no emotional or physical reaction will ever get the upper hand, or that the client will be able to remain surprisingly relaxed and strong while remembering things that would otherwise be stressful. If it proves necessary to work with the traumatic memories themselves, it is a good idea to decouple the normal stress responses which occur when remembering the relevant events from the stressful memories themselves, or to couple these memories with new relaxed responses. "Only go where it is safe" and "Relax and think about the bad things" can be used to lay the groundwork for an approach of this kind.

The client can be encouraged to focus on resource-related experiences, and to link these experiences with more and more aspects of the stressful memories or longer and longer periods of remembering. Sight, hearing and emotional state can be worked on separately in each case, and the client will become able to remember what he or she experienced for increasingly long periods of time.

The impact of the stressful memories can be weakened by using signal words to dissociate them, for example:

- time (past, i.e. "previous" memory),
- location (somewhere else, i.e. a memory you've had "until now"),
- person (third person, i.e. the memory of "your inner archivist"),
- verb (modal, i.e. "potential" memories that you "might have had"),

- level of reality (the memory "as you describe it"), or
- abstraction (i.e. "symptoms" instead of "pain").

The desired dissociative effect can be heightened as necessary by combining several such signal words.

An alternative approach is to reinforce the impact of resources by connecting them with concepts such as "here," "now," "you" and "I," making them more concrete and perceptible on a sensory and emotional level, and linking them with the dissociated stressful memories on this basis. A high proportion of the greetings in this book use this method (dissociation from stressful experiences and identification with liberating experiences through the use of signal words), and the effect achieved can be reviewed and stabilised using the greeting "The before-and-after test" from the section on trauma.

Stressful memories can be dissociated from the experience of "self," "here," "present" and "now," and moved from concrete existence and reality to reported reality; they can also be differentiated from each other or split up, i.e. divided into segments, and then fragmented yet further into smaller units which are easier to handle.[2]

In addition to dissociating stressful memories from the experience of self and from each other, and associating liberating experiences with each other and with the experience of self – and strengthening their internal plausibility and coherence – it is also possible to dissociate stressful experiences using inner films. Well-known and oft-discussed approaches in this context include the "cinema technique," which involves the trauma sufferer watching himself or herself from the outside while he or she views a film of the events, and the "strongbox exercise," during which the client locks the memories in an imaginary strongbox. The interventions "The father in your head" and "Journey to heaven" outline other methods for externalising stressful experiences through the use of film.

Only go where it is safe

T: **Fear, shame, feelings of guilt, trauma, anger**
R: **The unconscious**
M: **Your body can provide the ideal conditions for therapy by ensuring that all emotions and bodily reactions are well regulated at all times. It will not allow anything to get the upper hand.**

Please tell your unconscious that we are only going to travel to places where you feel safe and comfortable – we are *not* going to travel to places where you might experience fear or numbness. That's not the kind of emotions we need here! Can you pass on the message to your unconscious? Do you think it will be fine with that?[3]

As a general rule, use of this or a similar greeting at the start of a trauma therapy session is enough to avoid the client responding by withdrawing into numbness or experiencing violent abreactions.

Nothing will get the upper hand

T: **Trauma**
R: **The mind**
M: **Your body can ensure that every sensation and reaction is well regulated.**

Can we agree with your mind that whichever routes we travel down when we are talking with each other, nothing will ever get the upper hand – no emotion and no bodily reaction – and that everything will stay within a range which is comparatively pleasant for you and with which you are comfortable?

The greeting is suitable for use in all contexts, and is particularly useful when working with past trauma. It can be used alongside with the previous greeting or as a replacement.

Relax when thinking about the bad things

T: **Fear, shame, feelings of guilt, trauma, anger**
R: **The mind**
M: **If you ask it to, your mind can recondition itself within a matter of seconds, and produce pleasant or less unpleasant feelings in response to memories which used to be stressful.**

Send a greeting to your mind, and ask it to make sure that you can think with remarkable calm and even feelings of positivity about things you have probably regarded as extremely unpleasant so far. Your mind will be able to do what you ask. It will probably say, "Of course I can do it – why didn't you ask me before?"[4]

The greeting can be used instead of or as well as the two previous greetings, and any of them can be followed up with "The before-and-after test" in the interests of verifying and reinforcing the impact of therapy.

The before-and-after test

T: **Trauma**
R: **The mind**
M: **Your brain is already very good at keeping you calm while you remember stressful situations, and it can get even better at this task.**

Please tell me once again about the situation which use to cause you so much stress, so that we can see how well your brain is responding to the greeting we just sent it. . . . If I can share my observations, it seems to me that your forehead is smoother, your breathing is much deeper and more uniform, your voice is more resonant, and your speech is more fluent. . . . Send a greeting to your brain and say that it's doing a great job, and that from now on it should work on ensuring that you can think in an even more relaxed way about the things which used to cause you stress.[5]

The reconditioning is stabilised and reinforced by making the client aware of the alteration in his or her responses to memories which used to be stressful.

The father in your head

T: **Borderline (BPD), family, violence, abuse, trauma, neglect**
R: **The head and the internal image of the father**
M: **You do not need a solution which involves your actual father; a solution is possible which only involves your internal image of him, and this solution can work.**

> I'm not interested in your real father; he's not here, and even you only see the man himself rarely. I'm more interested in the image which you hold of him in your head, and which causes you stress on a daily basis even though your father is not physically present. Could we please take that father out of your head and sit him down over there?

Once there has been a shift from a landscape in which the client exists alongside the father to a landscape in which the father exists within the client, i.e. once the external and internal have been reversed in terms of the client's experience, he or she will feel capable of taking action rather than powerless.

Making a clear distinction between the physical father and the internal image of this father results in stress-relieving dissociation when discussing memories of him, and it soon becomes clear that the internal father (unlike the physical father) lies completely within the control of the client's mind.

Removing a violent father from one's head is a very different experience to bringing him into the room in one's imagination, even if he ends up sitting on the same chair in both instances. The former serves to relieve stress, while the latter can be unbearable.

Journey to heaven

T: **Borderline (BPD), family, violence, abuse, shame, feelings of guilt, trauma, neglect**

R: **Internal image of the father**

M: **Out of respect for yourself and others, you can use the cartoon technique to give the story a better and perhaps even a happy ending, regardless of whether or not that reflects the reality you have experienced to date.**

> Imagine telling your father that we will all die, and that once he has died he will meet many loving and wise people on the journey up to heaven, and that this experience will change him whether he wants it to or not. After returning from a 100-year trip full of encounters of this kind, what do you think he might say to you and what might he do, and how do you think things might have changed?

Framing the intervention in such a way that the client is invited to search for far-reaching changes in the father who exists in his or her head – without in any way detracting from the suffering he or she has endured at this father's hands – can lead to spectacular changes in the way that memories are handled. Clients with whom such an intervention has been used often report positive changes in relationships with the other members of their family, including the person who inflicted the original trauma.

Mania

The defining feature of mania is a delusional tendency to overestimate one's own capabilities and opportunities, coupled with exuberance, over-activity and (in most cases) a singular experience of meaning and happiness.

Questions such as "How long has that been the case? And what was going on when it happened for the first time?" often prompt reports of highly stressful events, which suggests that mania might be a response to traumatic experiences. In my opinion, the enormous amount of energy which goes into maintaining a manic phase serves to repress painful experiences which might be too much emotionally for the sufferer to bear.

Although a manic state can be experienced as pleasant at a subjective level, it consumes a great deal of energy, which leaves the sufferer at high risk of depression during the period of exhaustion which follows, when the stores of energy have run out. Although mania often morphs into depression, the reverse – depression morphing into mania – is not common.

As a fundamental principle, people in a manic state are blocking out painful aspects of reality. The good intention behind mania is presumably to cover up things which are too painful to think about by means of an existential construct which positions the client as a creative force rather than a victim, and by means of intense and pleasant stimuli and impulses which distract the sufferer from any painful memories. The greeting "A soft landing" both supports and undermines this suppression of reality, following the same principle as the paradoxical command not to think about a particular colour.

A soft landing

T: **Mania, psychosis, schizophrenia, grief, trauma, delusion**

R: **The mind**

M: **Congratulations on entirely forgetting all the bad things that have happened! If you find that you no longer have the energy you need to keep on forgetting them, make sure that your landing in whatever follows is a soft one.**

> You've already overcome so much – your life has not always been easy, but you've made it this far, and somehow you've coped with all the terrible things that have come your way, And now things are going well for you – perhaps even very well. Pass on my congratulations to your mind, and tell it that it does not need to remember all your earlier stressful experiences or to grieve them. It's great that you have so much energy, but if you should run out of steam at some point in the future, take care to make a soft landing – a soft and gentle landing.

The invitation to make a "soft landing" is an attractive proposition for the conscious mind, ensuring that the client does not put up any internal resistance; at the same time, however, it contains an instruction to the unconscious mind to avoid a crash landing at the end of the manic phase.

Depression

Someone suffering from depression is in a state of numbness, hopelessness and exhaustion, which in my opinion is closely related to traumatic experiences of powerlessness.

If you ask a sufferer of depression how long the depressive episodes – or the symptoms which can be interpreted as their precursors – have been going on, and what was happening around the time that they first emerged, sufferers typically report experiences of grieving alone, feeling unwelcome and being humiliated or excluded from a group. A common motif is a lack of community and support, and the good intention pursued by depression may be to replace the acute pain caused by such stressful experiences with an absence of feeling.

It is a singular fact that people suffering from depression often spend little time thinking about the events which appear to have triggered their symptoms, but are instead preoccupied with key questions of religion, morality, society and ecology. Reminding them of the presumed source of their depression can trigger grief, but this grief is often associated with a sense of relief – they find comfort in the idea that their suffering has a readily understandable cause rather than stemming from the all-perplexing problems to which it was previously attributed.

People suffering from depression behave as though they have a filter inside them which keeps out everything which might give them hope, encouragement or a sense of positivity, and depression-influenced communication can be described as the rejection of all possible life choices. Communicating with inner sceptics is therefore a vital aspect of working with depressive clients; they must be welcomed and praised for their good intentions, but they must also be dissociated from the self, assigned other tasks and transformed into persons performing a different role.

The greetings "Sceptics as external observers" and "Sceptics as guardians against disappointment" are good examples of this approach.

A very effective way of reducing the severity of depressive symptoms within a short period of time is described in "Greeting to the sleeping self" in the section on sleep problems. Reconditioning sleeping behaviours in such a way that the sufferer of depression falls more deeply asleep at the very first indications of a night-time awakening can allow him or her to sleep through the night within a matter of days; it is apparently the case not only that depression causes insomnia, but also that insomnia plays a large part in sustaining depression. A client's sense of well-being typically improves significantly and with long-lasting effect in the days following an intervention of this kind.

Sceptics as external observers

T: **Depression, scepticism**
R: **The sceptic within you**
M: **The people who exist within you and who object can be transformed into people who exist outside you, from commentators into observers, and from naysayers into discerning critics.**

Somewhere deep down inside you there might be someone who is sceptical about what we are doing here and about whether it will help you, and perhaps even about whether anything will ever help you at all. Send a greeting to this person, and pass on a request from me to go and stand over there, watch carefully and decide whether what we are doing is helpful.

Therapy is more effective in people suffering from depression and others with a habit of raising objections if their attitude of dissent can be weakened as early on in the process as possible.

Sceptics as guardians against disappointment

T: **Borderline (BPD), depression, scepticism**
R: **The sceptic within you**

M: **The sceptic within you wants to protect you against disappoint-ment. It has good reasons for doing so, and there's no reason why it shouldn't continue with this task. If we travel down paths which the sceptic has previously avoided, it's only because we are helping it to do its job.**

> I can well imagine that the person within you who feels so scepti-cal has suffered enough disappointment in life, and doesn't want to experience any more. Please tell your inner sceptic that we can work together – I don't want you to be disappointed again, and I'm sure that you don't either.

Inner sceptics can be interpreted as manifesting the client's desire – based on previous experiences – to avoid further disappointment. Instead of send-ing them away, it is a good idea to invite them to collaborate on the task of preventing disappointment. This intervention should preferably be followed by greetings to the inner sceptic which suggest ways in which the previ-ous attempts to protect the client against disappointment can be made more effective; examples include "Turning the sceptic into a silent observer" and "The Minister for Confidence" from the section on the effectiveness of therapy.

Exploiting the paradox of scepticism

T: **Depression, scepticism**
R: **The sceptic within you**
M: **If you have so far achieved the opposite of what you intended, now do the opposite of what you have done so far – perhaps that way you will achieve what you intend.**

> I think it's good news that you have an inner sceptic who protects you against disappointment. The only problem is that it accidentally – through its objections – causes the very disappointment it wants to prevent. Since your inner sceptic has good intentions, regardless of how clumsily it tries to implement them, I'd like to ask it to refrain from making objections for a few weeks, just as an experiment, and

perhaps even to boost your confidence and observe whether this is a more successful way of preventing disappointment.

The greeting can be expanded to include other comments and questions: "The person who has been sceptical up until now understands that too, and is perhaps simply looking for a way to do things differently," or "Do you think that the person who has raised objections up until now will agree to that?"

Freed from the ice

T: **Depression, grief, trauma**
R: **The mind**
M: **Once the numbness of depression has receded, painful feelings can bubble up to the surface. The inner self can regulate them in such a way that depression is no longer necessary as an emergency response to excessive pain.**

Imagine that you are a ship which got trapped in pack ice but is now free. You begin to rock backwards and forwards on the waves again, and now and then some spray comes over the bow. Tell your mind that it's all part of travelling by sea, and nothing unusual; and tell your mind that it should regulate the swell of the waves in such a way that you can always handle this rocking back and forth without too much effort, and don't need to worry about getting trapped in pack ice again.

The greeting has proven successful in helping people to return from the numbness of a depressive experience into the world of feelings, hope and self-experience.

Warming one's feet at the fire

T: **Depression, trauma**
R: **The mind**
M: **It can be painful for a short while when the numbness first passes, but after that is when things start to get better.**

> Your mind knows what it is like to come home after a long winter walk, with feet that are numb from cold and have no feeling in them. It also knows that it will hurt briefly when you start to warm your feet up by the fire. It knows that this is only a transitional phase; soon the feet will have thawed out, and then they will be warm.

A recovery from depression can often be accompanied by grief or pain of a different kind; learning to distinguish this experience from the depression itself and to interpret it as the first indications of a new zest for life can assist the recovery process. The greeting can be used to encourage clients not to flee from this state of pain back into the numbness of depression, but instead to move through the pain towards a new version of themselves, which allows them to experience well-being.[6]

Compulsive behaviour (OCD), tics, stuttering

If someone attempts to embody his or her key values in every aspect of his or her life – i.e. always to do and think certain things, and never to do and think others – certain other values may be neglected, and find expression in the form of strong counter-impulses.

Someone who believes passionately that it is wrong to commit acts of violence against others might suffer from a compulsive urge to commit exactly those acts. Someone with strong religious values might suffer from a compulsive urge to curse God, while at the same time believing that such behaviour condemns him or her to the fires of eternal damnation. Compulsive behaviour of this kind can occur whenever impulses (motivated by self-preservation or the need to express feelings, needs or sexuality) are forbidden, suppressed, regulated and controlled.

Compulsive thinking and compulsive action (or compulsive inaction, for example in the case of mutism) typically stem from an effort to impose deliberate control over impulses which are normally regulated involuntarily, such as feelings and thoughts.

In case after case, sufferers turn out to be afraid of something terrible happening because of their past or future guilt (because they have performed or will perform a prohibited action, or because they have failed or will fail to carry out a required action).

Tics can arise as a result of the sufferer's attempts to avoid experiencing or showing feelings, and his or her corresponding efforts to control and suppress the feelings or their expression.

In my view, Tourette syndrome functions as an extension of obsessive-compulsive or tic disorder; the sufferer's attempts to control and suppress expressions of feelings lead to them bursting out in an increasingly uncontrolled manner, which in turn means that the sufferer steps up his or her efforts to control them.

I have observed an ambivalence in people who stutter between the desire to take up as little time, space and attention as possible (perhaps for the benefit of *other* people in particular), and a countervailing desire to feel welcome and important, and to carve out space and time for themselves. In my opinion, both sides of this ambivalence should be given their due. It is important not to play them off against each other by simply demanding "fluid" speech (or in other words "do not take up too much time and attention"), but to work with the client to find other ways of remaining true to both values – perhaps by setting the dual goal of achieving recognition (by himself or herself and by others) of his or her intrinsic value while also taking a step back to allow other people to step forwards. "Adjust the clock" is a good example of an intervention of this kind.

Good intentions on both sides

T: **Stuttering, Tourette syndrome, compulsive behaviour (OCD)**
R: **The good intentions behind violent fantasies, the good intentions behind conflict avoidance**
M: **Both sides have good intentions, and these good intentions have a right to exist.**

Let's imagine that there are two people inside you – the one who comes up with all these violent fantasies, and the one who wants to avoid violence at all costs, who desires harmony and hates violence. And let's imagine that these people leave your body, and the one who likes violence stands over here on the left, and the one who likes harmony stands over here on the right. We can leave the undistilled violence and the undistilled harmony outside you, but let's send a greeting to the good intentions of both of these people, and tell them that they can return – the one on the left who demands the right to defend himself or herself, to live passionately and with energy and to take up space, and the one on the right who embodies the desire to belong, to be accepted and to be loved unconditionally. Now they are returning – how does that feel?

Obsessive-compulsive disorders can be interpreted as an ambivalence between certain values (e.g. accepting others) which are adhered to passionately, and other values (e.g. asserting oneself) which stand in conflict with the former, and are therefore suppressed – only to burst free with alarming force. Each of these two values are personified and dissociated from the experience of self, and the good intentions of both are then recognised and brought back into the self. The vehement exclusion of one value by the other is distinguished from the good intentions and "left outside" metaphorically speaking, or in other words removed from the experience of self.

The intervention can also be used for stuttering, in which case the two sides of the ambivalence can be described as demanding space, time and attention on the one hand, and allowing others to go first without standing in their way on the other.

Until the end of the universe

T: **Perfectionism, compulsive behaviour (OCD)**
R: **The seeker of perfection**
M: **Imagine that the symptoms are standing in personified form in front of you, that the residual symptoms of these symptoms are standing next to them, and that the residual symptoms of these residual symptoms are standing next in line, and so on and so on, into infinity!**

Imagine that there is someone inside you who loves completeness and perfection, and ask him or her to stand next to you and act as a quality manager. Now imagine that there is someone else inside you who suffers from compulsive thoughts, and stand him or her over here opposite you. Now that we've done that, we can put the person inside you suffering from any remaining compulsive thoughts alongside the first sufferer, and the person inside you with the remnants of these remaining compulsive thoughts next in the line. . . . Send a greeting to the person who loves completeness, and ask him or her to take over and continue putting the people with compulsive thoughts – or with the remnants of the remnants of the last remaining compulsive thoughts – in a line, one alongside another, right through the Milky Way until the end of the universe. . . .

This intervention has proven successful for clients or situations characterised by a particular focus on ambition, by a desire for security or perfection or by compulsive thoughts, and it frequently results in an immediate improvement in symptoms and continued improvements over the following hours, days and weeks.[7] The greeting can therefore also be used to counteract the loss of therapeutic effect in the period following a therapy session, as described in the section on improving therapeutic outcomes (for example the greeting "Only 90%").

Adjust the clock

T: **Work efficiency, burnout, music (rehearsing for performances), sports (performance optimisation), stuttering, compulsive behaviour (OCD)**

R: **The internal clock can be adjusted to a fast setting for the person inside you who wants to take up as little space, time and attention as possible, and to a very slow setting for the person inside you who would like to be as careful and thorough as possible.**

> Our brain can experience exactly the same period of time as passing either very rapidly or very slowly, as though there were an internal clock inside us whose hands can be adjusted to turn at a snail's pace or at the speed of light. The clock can be set to an extra slow setting for the person within you who is careful and thorough, and to a faster setting for the person who wants to take up as little space as possible. What would it feel like if you gave everyone his or her own clock, and if you gave a very slow-running clock to the person within you who has been stressed and impatient up until now?

Stuttering can be interpreted as a form of obsessive-compulsive disorder in which the client (as noted previously) is caught between two different goals: wanting to take up as little time and attention as possible (driven by a desire to take care of others, to avoid problems, to stick to the "house rules" or simply to belong), and wanting to be as thorough and careful as possible (for the same reasons, or as a counter-impulse motivated by self-preservation and self-care) – which takes time and attention.

The greeting can also be used for other problems relating to effective time management, avoiding inaccuracies and dealing with mistakes appropriately.

Delusion and psychosis

Psychosis sufferers frequently mention stressful situations they experienced in their childhood, and appear to have learned from these situations how to flee involuntarily into an intense and enduring dream world in order to escape a stressful reality. The events which bring on a psychotic episode are often similar to these original events and therefore act as traumatic triggers.

A striking feature of the events which bring on episodes of drug-induced psychosis is that they tend to occur before the phase of excessive drug consumption rather than before the psychosis which accompanies the subsequent withdrawal; in my opinion, drug use and psychosis both represent attempts to numb emotional pain, and the prescription of psychiatric drugs serves as a third alternative. In the long term, however, stresses of this kind can only be reduced and resolved by using trauma therapy methods and by teaching clients how to perceive and tolerate emotional pain and regulate it automatically.

The following section outlines a number of ideas for ways in which "greetings" can be incorporated into the treatment of schizophrenic disorders.

Dream mode

T: **Mania, psychosis, schizophrenia, trauma, delusion**
R: **The part of the mind which likes to dream**
M: **Your mind uses dreams to protect you from pain, and this is a good thing.**

   Instead of switching to dream mode whenever you experience reality, your mind can pinpoint the painful aspects of this reality, filter them out and transform them into a dream world.

A long, long time ago, back when you were a child, life was so difficult for you that you learned to dream very deeply, and the dream world became reality for you for extended periods of time. Whenever you are unwillingly reminded of something from back then, your mind is able to switch to this mode again. Send a greeting to your mind, and congratulate it on doing such a good job. Tell it that it could do an even better job by pinpointing the elements of your waking reality which are painful and replacing them with a dream world, rather than switching everything to dream mode. As it gets better at doing this, it should concentrate on pinpointing the painful parts of your waking reality with ever-increasing accuracy, and only replacing these parts with dreams.

As a general rule, psychosis sufferers are happy to discuss their dream world provided that you accept it as a good thing rather than trying to talk them out of their dreams. It is therefore more effective to assign value to the dream world and promote its role of preventing the acute pain associated with waking reality as experienced by the sufferer, rather than to attempt a wholesale reduction in psychotic experiences.

Core competencies

T: **Mania, psychosis, schizophrenia, trauma, delusion**
R: **The dream world**
M: **If the world around you is exactly the same as it was when you first entered your dream world, please keep on dreaming; if not, it's time to restock the shelves.**

> Tell your dream world that it should keep on covering up reality for you whenever you are faced with a situation which is exactly the same as it was back then when life was so hard for you. Ask it to make sure that what happened to you back then never happens again – which means that it only needs to switch to dream world mode if exactly the same people who were present back then are doing exactly the same things as they did back then. Everything else should be removed from the "dream world shelf," as if it were food past its sell-by date. Would your dream world be happy to focus on its core competencies in this way?

This greeting has a similar structure to the previous one, with the difference that the focus shifts from protecting oneself against the pain itself (instead of the totality of the waking reality in which the pain is experienced) to the pain experienced in a situation which is exactly the same as the original event which triggered the escape into a dream world (instead of situations which merely have parallels with the traumatic situation).

The fastest way to get out is to keep up the good work!

T: **Psychosis, schizophrenia, delusion**
R: **The dreaming self**
M: **Feel free to keep on dreaming – but try to dream better so that you can leave the closed ward as soon as possible.**

> Send a greeting to your dreaming self, and ask it to continue doing such a good job of looking after you. It simply needs to work a little bit harder so that we can get you out of the closed ward as soon as possible and make sure that you don't end up back here again in future. Would your dreaming self agree to that?[8]

The greeting contains a therapeutic double bind;[9] it expressly supports the psychotic behaviour of the client's unconscious mind, while at the same time suggesting that this experience should be modified in such a way that the client no longer needs to stay on a closed ward.

To each his own

T: **Psychosis, schizophrenia, delusion**
R: **The mind**
M: **You can keep your dreaming self, but sometimes it must step to one side so that the waking self (which experiences what is referred to as reality by the people surrounding you) can take over and act in your best interests.**

> In order to avoid worrying the hospital staff and the judge, it's important that you keep as much of the dream world as *you* need, while at the same time noticing as much of what is going in waking reality as the other people around you do. That will allow you to interact with these others not from the perspective of your dreaming self, but from the perspective of the waking reality which is all they understand. Send a greeting to your mind, and ask it to ratchet up the waking self and ratchet down the dreaming self whenever you talk to these people.[10]

When asked about their childhood, many psychosis sufferers report that they were forced to escape into another world mentally (since they could not do so physically) as a result of violence inflicted by family members. In my opinion, therefore, psychosis is a response to traumatic stresses, or in other words to being overwhelmed by feelings of powerlessness. Although a stay on a closed ward can be an understandable consequence of psychotic episodes, it often gives rise to an experience of powerlessness similar to that which originally (and perhaps repeatedly thereafter) triggered the psycho-sis. Psychosis sufferers undergoing in-patient treatment are therefore often preoccupied not only with the main focus of their mania but also with a desire to be discharged from hospital.

The greeting contains two therapeutic double binds. Firstly, it suggests that the client can keep his or her dreaming self (or in other words the psy-chotic experience), with the underlying assumption that he or she can some-times reduce the intensity of these dreams. Secondly, it praises the dreaming self for reducing the client's pain while at the same time proposing that the client could temporarily return to the reality experienced by other people in order to escape detention (and the retraumatising experience of confine-ment) as soon as possible.

Both dream world and waking world

T: **Psychosis, schizophrenia, delusion**
R: **The part of the mind that knows what is real for everyone, the dreaming self (two recipients for two messages)**
M: **Make sure that enough of the reality experienced by everyone else is available to all parts of your mind when you interact with others so that they can't find reasons to detain you. You can continue to use dreams as a way of promoting inner happiness.**

Ask the part of your mind that knows what is real for everyone to make sure that it always has enough of the reality experienced by eve-ryone else in order to interact with them at this level of reality, so that they are no longer worried about you and agree to discharge you. Your dreaming self is welcome to keep on producing the dreams which you need to be happy, but it should make sure that there is always enough reality left over for you to engage in conversations with other people. Do you think that will work?[11]

The double bind in this greeting is actively framed as a double dissocia-tion of two inner persons that are addressed in parallel rather than being placed above and below each other in a hierarchy. An additional (hierarchi-cal) dissociation is established between the "mind" and "part of the mind." However the primary distinction made by the greeting is between two parts of the person on the one hand, and the person himself or herself on the other; "you," the "part of your mind who knows what is real for everyone" and the "dream self."

Before the dream becomes a nightmare

T: **Psychosis, schizophrenia, delusion**

R: **The part of the mind that knows what is real for everyone**

M: **At the very first indication that pleasant dreams are turning into nightmares, switch to "reality as it is experienced by everyone" as a preferable alternative to the world of nightmares.**

The part of you who is responsible for knowing what is real for everyone else can watch out for signs that your world of helpful dreams is turning into a world of harmful nightmares, and introduce a bit of reality at the very first indication that this is happening. Send a greeting to the part of you who is familiar with "reality as it is experienced by everyone else," and ask him or her to do this for you.[12]

This intervention is similar to other greetings which are used to recondition abnormal sleeping behaviours such as difficulty sleeping at night because of depression or grief, or sleep apnoea.[13] At the first indication that a pleasant dream might be turning into a nightmare as a result of psychosis, the inner person who knows what is real for everyone else should intervene and return the client to a state of waking reality.

Dreaming and waking – do more of the same!

T: **Psychosis, schizophrenia, delusion**

R: **The dreaming self, the part of the mind that knows what is real for everyone (two recipients and two messages)**

M: **The dreaming self should dream more, and the waking self should wake up more.**

Send a greeting to your dreaming self and to the person within you who knows what is real for everyone else, and ask them to keep on doing what they are already doing but to do it even better, and to make sure that you always have enough "reality" available outside your dream world for your own requirements and for the other people you encounter.[14]

This greeting contains a double bind, since it promotes both sides of an ambivalence – symptomatic behaviour which makes it impossible to build relationships with others on the one hand, and symptom-free behaviour which might allow relationships to be built (but may also lead to threatening encounters) on the other. Since the greeting welcomes the dreaming self rather than fighting it, the latter does not experience a compulsive need to keep on dreaming. The more that dreaming is encouraged, the less waking reality appears to be a threat. The idea that psychotic experiences offer a form of protection makes the sufferer more open to non-psychotic experiences; the waking self can be awake more because the dreaming self is able to dream more.

A new operating system

T: **Psychosis, residual schizophrenia, delusion, postoperative delirium**

R: **The brain**

M: **Your brain can identify the remnants of psychosis which do not fit with the rest of what you are experiencing, and adjust them or replace them with something else which fits with the vast majority of what you are experiencing as reality.**

> Switching from psychosis to a state of normality is like switching between two different operating systems – Windows and Linux, for example. Send a greeting to your brain, and suggest that a few bugs might pop up in the programs and functions running on the new operating system. Ask it to scan the hard drive and replace the relevant files or add new ones, for as long as necessary.[15]

This greeting is designed for clients who spend most of their time in a non-psychotic state, but still occasionally fall prey to delusional ideas. It can be used in a similar form for people who are experiencing postoperative delirium or brief reactive psychosis and find it difficult to come to terms with reality.

Grief

Grief occurs in response to the loss of a person or (in the broader sense of the word) the loss of an object, a hope, a belief, a group, an activity, an environment or an opportunity which previously gave the sufferer's life meaning or formed part of his or her identity.

If identity means getting to know my image as it is reflected back to me from the mirror of the important people in my life and how they see and treat me, the loss of one of these people also signifies a loss in terms of the way that I experience my identity. Grief means that my inner self is looking for a way to come to terms with both an external and an internal loss.

The difficulty of influencing the grieving process is readily apparent, and the question as to whether an attempt to do so should be made in a therapeutic setting is a valid one.

Nevertheless, grief often has a detrimental impact on people's health and their ability to maintain social relationships, or even to drive safely on the roads. Grieving also places people at a higher risk of developing an addiction, and grief can sometimes turn into depression or a similar chronic mental illness.

The burden of grief can be reduced enormously if the sufferer can shift his or her attention away from what has been lost, and towards something associated of value which remains or is just beginning. This is the approach followed in the greeting "The invisible second half."

In addition, sufferers often experience a significant reduction in grief if they are able to accept its ambivalence and distinguish between the value of the grief itself and the strategies which their body has come up with to express this value (with the associated side effects). This suggestion is embodied in the greeting "The magnitude of pain and the magnitude of love."

The invisible second half

T: **Imprisonment, migration, grief**
R: **The inner self**
M: **The life you shared continues, just in a different way.**

When someone dies, we think that they have gone away – but in fact they keep on living within us. If it seems like a good idea to you, tell your inner self that what began back then was the invisible second half of your life together.

The last sentence of this greeting should be voiced slowly, carefully and with particular emphasis in order to underline its importance. Although many might disagree, it is possible and healthy to find continuity and community with a loved one even after his or her death. If we shift our attention from what has been left behind in the past to what remains and what is now beginning, keeping the person we loved at the centre of our attention as we do so, the nature of our grief changes. The message embodied in this greeting is received by many clients with relief and gratitude.

The magnitude of pain and the magnitude of love

T: **Imprisonment, grief, separation, feeling unwelcome, loss**
R: **Grief**
M: **The amount of pain you feel is not a measure of your love or loyalty, or of your striving for constancy and belonging. It can be regulated independently of these values.**

> Send a message to your grief, and tell it that the magnitude of your love does *not* need to be a measure of the magnitude of your pain. It is possible to have loved a lot and to stay true to all your values *without* suffering accordingly. Your inner self can distinguish the good intentions which lie behind your grief from your pain. How does that allow you to feel?[16]

The emotional stress endured by grieving clients can often be reduced significantly if we alert them to the fact that their inner self can regulate the experience of suffering and the experience of remaining true to values independently of each other.

What would your mother say about that?

T: **Grief, feelings of guilt**
R: **Mother (deceased)**
M: **The deceased are merciful. The person towards whom you feel guilty probably sees the situation differently. The more deeply you experience your loss, the more likely it is that your mother will be generous in her opinion of you. You should let her (or your internal film of her) interpret the situation, because she is the one most affected by it.**

> If we imagine that it is possible to visit the hereafter where your mother is, and if you were to visit her there and say to her, "Mother, the guilt for your death lies at my feet," how do you think she would answer you?

The more guilty the survivor of the deceased person feels, the more likely it is that he or she will view the mother as generous and value-driven. And if he or she tends to lend greater weight to the mother's rights and interests than to his or her own, it is likely that the mother's generous attitude will be deemed believable. The deceased's purported answer is generally something along the lines of, "Why on earth are you worrying about that? That's all in the past!" or "That's OK. Don't worry about me. I'm happy now." The following question can also be added: "Who could possibly know you better than your own mother?"

Passing on the legacy

T: **Grief**
R: **The deceased person**
M: **I will pass on to others the things which you passed on to me, just as you would have done. In this way you can continue to act through me, and I can show you my gratitude.**

> In your thoughts, send your mother a greeting and tell her than you will pass on to others all the good things that she passed on to you, just as she herself would undoubtedly have done. In this way your mother can continue doing good for the world through your heart, your mouth and your hands. By passing on the good she would have done, you are giving it back to your mother in the form of a thank-you gift.

The greeting suggests that it is possible to view the whole situation differently, and that the loving "give and take" which formerly took place between the client and the deceased can continue despite the latter's death.[17]

Greetings to my future child

T: **Disability, reproductive medicine, premature birth, pregnancy, still-birth, grief, trauma, twins (multiples)**
R: **Child in utero (embryo)**
M: **Part of me feels pain, but these feelings relate to another child, not you. It's important not to get confused.**

> Send a greeting to the child whom you are carrying within you, and tell him or her: you are unique and wonderful! And if you do sense

any fear or confusion within me, it has nothing to do with you, but with a completely different child, from a time before you came into being. You and this other child feature in two very different stories, which have nothing to do with each other.

The primary recipient of this greeting (and the recipient for whom it is really intended) is not the child, but the pregnant woman, who is told three things: It's only right for you to grieve one child. It's only right for you to be happy about the other child. Make sure that you differentiate between the two and match the right feeling to the right child.

A modified version of the greeting can also be used if a highly stressful event occurs shortly after a child is born – for example, a death (perhaps of a twin) or the separation of the parents.

Self-confidence and self-awareness

In order to build up an idea of who they are, small children look to the other people in their environment and the kind of treatment they receive from them. We all carry around internal images of these "other people" inside us, and they tell us what we are worth, or in other words how much self-confidence we have. Childhood experiences of feeling (or not feeling) that we belong and that we are welcome, loved and respected have an enormous impact on how self-confident we feel in later life.

An individual's level of self-confidence can vary between different areas of his or her life; he or she may feel confident at work but insecure about his or her gender identity, have mixed feelings about his or her domestic skills and a poor opinion of his or her artistic abilities.

It is tempting to think that the past is over and done with and cannot be changed, but memories are the only biologically relevant part of the past, and memories always take place in the present. Every time that we see, hear, feel or think something that reminds us of an earlier time, these triggers release an interconnected web of emotions, internal images and bodily reactions, but these conditioned responses – which are nothing other than memories – can be reshaped, and they include the ideas about ourselves that we repeatedly and involuntarily perpetuate when we think about our abilities, our idiosyncrasies and our intrinsic value.

It is often said that what has happened in the past cannot be altered, that something which has been present for a long time will take a long time to change and that symptoms which are thought to be severe can only be cured with difficulty. In my opinion, ideas such as these are detrimental when working with clients whose negative self-image was formed in childhood, and the following attitude is more helpful: "Everything which is relevant for your body takes place within it in the present, and can therefore also be altered and reshaped in the present."

Finding energy

T: **Anxiety, burnout, depression, motivation, compulsive behaviour (OCD)**
R: **The body**
M: **We can spontaneously know at any time what will help us or hinder us, and our bodily sensations will guide us.**

Send a greeting to your body, and ask it to provide you with detailed feedback on how it is feeling during every thought you think, during every word you say, and during everything you do: does it feel powerful, lively and full of energy, or listless, irritated and chaotic? Tell your body that you want to continue doing anything that makes you feel stronger and do more of it, and stop doing anything that makes you feel weaker or do less of it. Your body can help you with this task.

This greeting is suitable for use in a wide range of contexts.

Your best friend

T: **Aggression, borderline (BPD), burnout, depression, belief, help, perfectionism, self-confidence, compulsive behaviour (OCD)**
R: **The brain**
M: **If you find yourself being harsher on yourself than you would be on the people you love, stop yourself and try again.**

Do you sometimes berate yourself and hold yourself to higher standards than the other people around you? Make the following request from your brain: whenever you talk to yourself or treat yourself less kindly than you would talk to or treat your best friend, it can interrupt you and show you what it would look like if you were to talk to or treat yourself just as kindly. Then you can carry on with whatever you were thinking.

This greeting is also suitable for use in a wide range of contexts.

People who were not made to feel welcome when they were children, or those who experienced childhood neglect or violence, are at greater risk of treating themselves in the ways described here.

The ancestor who knows what's best for you

T: **Career, depression, family, self-confidence, self-value, feeling unwelcome**
R: **Someone feeling unsure of himself or herself (with a loving ancestor as the sender of the greeting)**
M: **Somewhere deep inside you is someone who knows exactly what you are good at and how capable you are, and he or she has good news for anyone who has doubted you in the past. See for yourself, and be amazed at the results!**

Imagine that one of your many millions of ancestors – one who knows exactly why you are a good and valuable person – leaves the imaginary confines of your head and faces someone else who has also left these imaginary confines, the person within you who disagrees with this assessment. Listen to what the ancestor who loves you is telling this person. What kind of surprises do you think he or she might have in store?

If the client finds it difficult to imagine what the ancestor might say, it is a good idea to start by asking him or her to describe the bodily posture that might be assumed by this loving person, and how this person might look, sound and breathe. Then the client can put himself or herself in the ancestor's shoes, and tune into his or her inner impulses to identify the good things the loving ancestor might want to tell the inner person who is less sure.

Fear of speaking in public and exam nerves

Fear of speaking in public and exam nerves are not necessarily linked to a general lack of self-confidence; in many cases, they can be traced back to specific biographical experiences which resulted in exams or other experiences of putting oneself forwards being associated with failure or other stressful situations. The sufferer felt completely at the mercy of events, and lost all hope of being able to achieve a better result through behavioural changes.

Clients commonly respond in one of two ways if they are asked when they first experienced exam nerves, and what was going on in their lives at the time. Some talk about their experiences of grief, fear of loss or trauma, and others talk about unexpected punishments or failures which came in the place of anticipated praise and good marks. In my opinion, this suggests that exam nerves can arise in two different ways. In the first of these, grief or a different but similarly stressful situation results in an initial deterioration in performance; the original trigger is later forgotten, and the client comes to believe that he or she is "bad at exams," which becomes a self-fulfilling prophecy. The second way in which exam nerves can arise is when someone has revised hard but been rewarded for his or her efforts with an unexpected punishment, leaving him or her with the belief that revising hard will mean bad news in the long run.

The emergence of a fear of exams and failure is also more likely among people who tend to have high expectations of themselves and simultane-ously fail to acknowledge any progress and achievements they have made. By doing so, they are often copying the behaviour of a parental attachment figure, and the situation is complicated yet further if the child was led to believe that parental affection was dependent on academic success, if the recognition through which this affection was expressed was short in supply and if the chances of succeeding in this quest were uncertain. Sometimes clients find themselves faced with a curious double bind, as though they were torn between two competing camps: "I must do my absolute best in order to be loved" versus "even if I do my absolute best, I won't get much back."

Learning is playing

T: **Exam nerves, exam failure, school anxiety**
R: **The child you used to be**
M: **Take control! If you take control, revising for and passing exams will be no more difficult than playing with Lego.**

Back when you were a toddler aged just one or two, you learned to speak your native language quickly and easily, without any grades or exams. You learned to sit, stand, walk and run. You built things with Lego blocks, you played pirates and hide and seek and you learned to ride a bicycle; you overcame all of these hurdles and learned what you wanted to learn, as if by magic. Send a greeting to the child inside you and tell it to take control once again. Whenever you are learning or reading, whenever you are taking an exam and writing something on an exam paper or saying something to an examiner, in reality it is nothing more and nothing less than playing with Lego blocks.

In the past I had great success encouraging school pupils and university students suffering from exam nerves to adopt this attitude through the use of hypnosis proper. I now tend to use short greetings such as the one here, with a similarly high rate of success.

Investment

T: **Love triangle, migration, dating, exam nerves, starting up a company, compulsive behaviour (OCD), career**
R: **Someone who is hesitating**
M: **Investment means accepting a risk of failure in return for a chance of success.**

Send a greeting to the person inside you who is hesitating, and tell him or her that the way to the promised land leads over a narrow bridge. You will cross this bridge if your desire to get to the other side outweighs your fear of falling. Investment means saying yes to something you desire, and from the very outset accepting a risk of failure in return. Once you do that, you will find that the way forwards is clear.

This greeting works well with clients who are afraid of trying something new and therefore remain trapped in old structures which may no longer be appropriate. It can be particularly effective as a way of encouraging clients to move forwards if they are on the verge of embarking on new careers or entering new relationships.

Sleep

Common sleep disorders include difficulty falling asleep and remaining asleep, early waking, sleepwalking, nightmares and night terrors. Sending greetings to the unconscious mind is an extremely effective way of processing these problems and reconditioning sleep behaviours.

Greetings can also be used to solve problems such as teeth grinding, sleep apnoea, snoring and oversleeping.

"Greeting to the sleeping self" has proven particularly helpful when working with clients experiencing difficulty remaining asleep, especially those suffering from grief and depression.

Greetings can also be used to treat nocturnal bedwetting by children and adults in the absence of underlying organic causes. The last two greetings in this section provide examples of how this can be achieved.

Greeting to the sleeping self

T: **Burnout, depression, insomnia, grief, trauma**
R: **The sleeping self**
M: **You can identify the early indications of things that would previously have woken you up, and interpret them as prompts to sleep more deeply.**

Send a greeting to your sleeping self – tell it to notice whatever wakes you up, and to sleep *more deeply* whenever it notices the *early indications* that it is happening again. An interesting side effect might be that you feel less exhausted, which in turn reduces your symptoms of depression. Keep an eye on things until we see each other again, and tell me if you make any interesting findings.[18]

This greeting works very well with clients who are experiencing difficulty remaining asleep as a result of depression, grief or trauma, or because they have imposed a heavy schedule and workload on themselves. Certain people are prompted to wake up by the sleeping situation itself (deep sleep, a certain time, a certain bed, sleeping with other people in the house) because they experienced trauma at night, and it may be necessary to reverse this conditioning first in order to avoid the idea expressed in the greeting being vetoed by a "bodyguard." One way of achieving this might be with a greeting which contains an invitation only to wake up in the previous manner if exactly the same situation occurs as when the client first woke up in this way, with the same people in the same roles.

Sleep apnoea

T: **Sleep apnoea**
R: **The body**
M: **You can identify the early signs of interrupted breathing while you are asleep, and interpret them as a reminder to breathe deeply and regularly.**

> Send a greeting to your body, and tell it that from now on it should breathe particularly deeply at the *first sign* of interrupted breathing during the night, so that you can carry on sleeping even more peacefully than before.[19]

The outcome of this greeting is that weak and irregular breathing, tense muscles and fear are interpreted as a prompt to breathe particularly deeply and regularly, rendering phases of sleep apnoea unnecessary. The greeting can be framed with stories about how people learn to wake up and go to the bathroom in response to early warnings of nocturnal bedwetting (pressure in the bladder), how they learn to turn over in response to early signs of falling out of bed (one arm hanging over the edge of the bed), and how they learn to wake up one minute before the alarm clock because an internal clock alerts them to the time; all of these stories increase the likelihood that sleep behaviours will be conditioned.

Fear-free breathing

T: **Nightmares, postoperative delirium, brief reactive psychosis, comas, anaesthesia, (night-time) panic attacks, Parkinson's disease (side effect of medication), night terrors, trauma (traumatic event which occurred at night or which woke the victim from sleep), anxiety**
R: **The sleeping self**
M: **You can make a deal with your sleeping self to change anxious breathing into calm breathing.**

> Pass on this message to your sleeping self: while you're asleep, if you start to breathe in a way that might suggest that you're feeling anxious, it can cause you to breathe in long, deep, calm waves, and make these waves longer and longer, deeper and deeper, and calmer and calmer.[20]

This greeting is a good way of systematically reducing the client's level of anxiety while asleep (or under anaesthetic or in a coma), thereby reducing nightmares, night terrors and night-time panic attacks.

Alternatively, the following stimulus can be used: ". . . whenever the anxiety you feel in your dreams scores more than 2 out of 10 . . ."

The snoring angel

T: **Nightmares, night terrors, sleepwalking, snoring, teeth grinding**
R: **The snoring person**
M: **The snoring person can stand next to your bed at night, watch over you and relieve you of all the unnecessary physical and emotional tension which has previously made you snore.**

Before you fall asleep, imagine that you can remove from your body the person who often snores at night, and stand him or her next to your bed as a guardian angel. Ask your guardian angel to check up on you regularly while you sleep, and to take away any increased muscular tension or emotional stress; you can also hand over any tension or stress at regular intervals. Praise him or her if the job is done well and you snore less, and offer motivation if he or she needs to work a bit harder.

Alternatively, an inner person within whomever is sleeping alongside the snorer can be asked to sleep even more deeply every time that it hears the sound of snoring, or this person can send a greeting to the snorer telling it that "any sign of snoring from you is a signal for me to keep on breathing quietly." The greetings "Redistributing tension" and "Work on the rigging" from the section on the muscular system are also useful in this connection.[21]

Shut the floodgates!

T: **Enuresis**
R: **The bladder**
M: **Having a dry bed or a wet bed when you wake up in the morning is not simply something you have to endure passively, but a decision taken by the organs in your body, and you can encourage them to take the decision which suits you best.**

Send a greeting to your bladder, and ask it to keep the floodgates shut tonight.

This greeting was developed by a seminar participant when she was saying goodnight to her 11-year-old daughter one evening. Her daughter suffered from primary enuresis, but her bed was dry next morning (which was an unusual occurrence). The following morning brought another wet bed, so the seminar participant suggested the greeting below to her daughter that evening.

Turn off the tap!

T: **Enuresis**

R: **The kidneys, via the brain (two-level greeting)**

M: **It isn't you – or in other words your conscious mind – that needs to do the work, but your unconscious mind. Your body will work on your behalf as long as it is given the right instructions. Your body can solve the problem in several different ways.**

> Tell your brain to send a greeting to your kidneys, and ask them to produce less urine again tonight.

"That's just like in that song by the singer Otto Waalkes – 'big brain calling little brain!'" exclaimed the daughter, and laughed. No further conversations were necessary. The following morning the bed was dry again for the second time, and it remained dry for three out of the next four nights. Two months later, the mother told me that her daughter was completely dry at night for the first time in her life.

Food, addiction, habits

One way of reducing addictive behaviour is to dissociate (at the level of the imagination) the addict from the client who is physically present – for example, the client can be encouraged to place the invisible addict on a seat other than the one on which he or she is sitting, to examine and honour this addict's good intentions, and to suggest that cooperation might be a good way to remain truer to these good values in the future. The intervention "Supporting the smoker's good intentions" outlines an approach of this kind.

Another option is to ask the client to identify which areas of his or her life are highly controlled, disciplined and well-organised, and which are less so. He or she should then try to identify the advantages of both, and to think about the additional benefits that might arise if they were able to exist in harmony with each other. The therapy room can be divided into two different physical areas: a controlled half associated with success and recognition but also with effort, and an uncontrolled half associated with relaxation, pleasure or autonomy. The client can be asked to place himself or herself in the controlled half, to fill up an imaginary bucket with the benefits available on this side, and then to move over to the other, uncontrolled half of the room and observe any changes that occur. The client can then be asked to fill up his or her bucket with the benefits of the relaxed, autonomous, uncontrolled area of life, and to carry this experience back over to the controlled area of life and observe any changes that occur.[22] The distinction between the two different areas of life can then be eliminated, or a third area established which is independent of both of them. During this procedure, greetings can be sent to the disciplined inner person or the freedom-loving inner person, or to the person who the client will be once he or she has freed himself or herself from this constricting dichotomy.

The options outlined are aimed at dissociating the addict from the self or dissociating the addicted inner person and the disciplined inner person from each other and from the self, and then forming new and more helpful associations between these persons and between them and the self.

When working with clients suffering from anorexia, it is also possible to ask the hidden inner person who knows what a healthy weight and a healthy way of eating look like in reality to take control over the client's life, regardless of any conscious thoughts on these matters by the client or other people; this procedure is described in the greeting "A healthy weight."

Similar procedures can of course be used for other forms of addictive behaviour; instead of sending a greeting to an inner person who knows what a healthy weight looks like in reality, it is possible to call on the person within the mind who has a special and involuntary ability to regulate emotional pain, and more specifically the pain associated with experiences from the period when the addiction started.

A healthy weight

T: **Anorexia, bulimia, eating disorder, body dysmorphic disorder**
R: **The part of the unconscious mind that knows what a healthy weight looks like in reality**
M: **Adapt eating behaviours in a way which is likely to lead to a healthy weight, regardless of what the conscious mind thinks is right.**

I don't want to talk to you about whether you are underweight or overweight, and I'm sure you've had enough of these conversations yourself. If it's alright with you, I think we should talk to the part of your unconscious mind that knows better than you and better than my conscious mind what healthy eating and a healthy weight would *really* mean for you, and ask it to make any necessary changes to your eating behaviour from now on, regardless of who is right and who is wrong in these conversations. Would it be OK if we did that?

I developed this greeting while working with an anorexic patient; during the following session she reported that she couldn't understand it – she had put on weight, but she didn't mind.[23]

Supporting the smoker's good intentions

T: **Smoking, addiction**
R: **The part of you who sometimes smokes**
M: **You are pursuing good intentions, and I want to help you to achieve them!**

Send a greeting to the part of you who sometimes smokes. I know that he only wants the best for you – perhaps to reward you, comfort you or relax you. I think it would be a good idea to work together with him or her so that he or she can do an even better job of achieving these good intentions, without the previous side effects. Do you think he or she would agree? And how about you?[24]

Recognising and supporting the good intentions of the client's former inner smoker serves as a basis for encouraging the cooperation of inner persons who might otherwise pursue interests which stand at odds with the goal of therapy.

Immune system

The first intervention in this section is aimed at strengthening the immune system so that it can fight off infectious diseases; the following interventions can be used when working with clients who suffer from allergies, asthma and food intolerances, as well as other complaints such as Crohn's disease and colitis.

Allergic symptoms are disproportionately strong defensive reactions on the part of the body to triggers which are often relatively harmless. When clients suffering from allergies are asked when the symptoms first emerged, they regularly say that it was during a time of severe emotional stress – perhaps linked to a single event, to the confluence of several events, or to the reactivation of earlier traumatic experiences.

If the mind is asked to separate out the event which originally triggered the allergy and the allergic responses, or to identify them in such a way that the allergy only occurs when exactly the same trigger event is repeated, the allergy disappears. Different allergies can however relate back to different trigger events, meaning that the procedure may need to be repeated for the various allergic responses.

In terms of therapeutic procedure, I do not differentiate between allergies and food intolerances.

I regard allergies as an erroneous equivalence between the body's own defence systems and an external hazard, and the phenomenon has many similarities with a phobia in terms of its progression;[25] observable symptoms in the case of allergies include responses of the skin and the mucous membranes, whereas the defensive reactions in the case of a phobia consist of fear and disgust. The sufferer is caught in a vicious cycle in which defences are raised to counter the hazard, and these raised defences are misinterpreted as a sign of an even larger hazard. In case after case, it is possible to identify particular emotional stresses which were present at the time when the first symptoms of the disorder occurred and which triggered it; both allergies and phobias can therefore be regarded as post-traumatic stress responses.[26] Triggers can include individual events, a series of events or key stimuli originating from earlier traumatic events.

A good example can be found in the case of a woman suffering from lactose intolerance, who reported that she spat milk out with such disgust as a newborn that it was touch and go for several weeks as to whether or not she would survive. When asked to describe the circumstances of her birth, she explained that her mother had fallen pregnant as the result of an affair, and had been told by her partner in the affair that she should get an abortion; she ended the affair and returned to her husband, who accepted the baby as the price he had to pay to keep his wife, and who persuaded himself – despite knowing deep down that it was a lie – that she must be his daughter. When the woman realised that there was a link between the lactose intolerance and the circumstances of her birth, the symptoms disappeared.

The reverse infection

T: **Cold, flu, infection**
R: **Bacteria**
M: **If bacteria can infect humans, then the reverse is also true!**

> Send a greeting to the bacteria, and tell them that they should watch out and make sure that they don't get infected with Ruth (client's name) – because if they do, things will surely end badly for them!

The purpose of this greeting is to change a defensive attitude to an infection into an offensive one, thereby not only improving the client's sense of emotional well-being but also laying a better foundation for the body to defend itself against pathogens.

An infection – or an epidemic?!

T: **Cold, flu, infection**
R: **The immune system**
M: **If bad things like infections can spread, then so can good things!**

> I have infectious health. Send a greeting to your immune system, and tell it to watch out and make sure that it doesn't catch anything from me.

The intervention results in a reversal of attention on the part of the client; instead of concentrating on defending himself or herself against something he or she does not want, the focus is shifted towards perceiving and strengthening something he or she wants (resilience). It is highly unlikely that a statement such as this – which appears to be merely a joke – will be contradicted, and this is precisely why the mental placebo it contains can achieve the desired effects without encountering any obstacles.

The warning embodied in this greeting results in a counter-reaction. The listener internally disagrees with the command to be careful and "not to catch anything," and responds with an impulse to do exactly the opposite, i.e. "to catch something." This distracts the client's attention yet further from the idea that health cannot be infectious and any protests to this effect, thus increasing the effectiveness of the suggestion.[27]

Allergies and trauma

T: **Allergy,   asthma,   autoimmune   disease,   food   intolerance, neurodermatitis**
R: **An allergy**

M: **Feel free to keep on fighting the pollen, but only when you are in the same stressful situation as you were when the symptoms first occurred.**

> Allergies often begin in the same way as a post-traumatic stress disorder; during a period of emotional overload, you develop a defence response to triggers which are harmless in reality. Send a greeting to your allergy, and tell it that it is welcome to keep on fighting the pollen, but only if you are in *exactly* the same stressful situation as you were when the symptoms first occurred.

The intervention belongs to the "retraining bodyguards" category:[28] the conditioned response is supported and differentiated rather than fought against.

Confusing two problems

T: **Allergy, cold**
R: **The immune system**
M: **Don't worry about allergies – worry about fighting off infections!**

> Sometimes if you have a cold, it can be difficult to tell which symptoms are part of the cold and which are part of an allergy – and your body might mistakenly fire up the defences against pollen even though it should really be worrying about viruses. Send a greeting to your immune system, and tell it that there must have been a misunderstanding; it should worry about fighting off infections instead of worrying about allergies.

This model also explains why allergies tend to increase in severity during periods of mental stress. If the body does not know exactly what it ought to be fighting, sometimes it chooses to defend itself against substances that were particularly in evidence during the period of stress rather than against a complex or existentially hazardous threat to the psyche.

Muscular system

Muscular tension is experienced as increased tension in certain parts of the body; the natural corollary of this is that decreased tension is experienced in other parts of the body. Sending greetings to both the over-stressed and the under-stressed muscles can offer a new perspective on the situation which can help to dissipate the symptoms.

As a basic principle, it has proven helpful to address not only the muscles in the area of the body experienced consciously by the client as being directly affected, but the muscles throughout the entire body.

The same applies when working with clients who snore, and an intervention to this effect can be found in the section on sleep.

Redistributing tension

T: **Lumbago, muscular tension, snoring, torticollis**
R: **Muscles, networks of muscles**
M: **The under-stressed muscles should absorb stress and the over-stressed muscles should release stress, until the stress ratios in all the muscles throughout your body correspond to your inner model of correct muscular stress.**

Send a greeting to the muscles inside you which have so far been under less stress than intended, and tell them to increase their level of stress and to relieve the burden on the muscles which temporarily helped out by taking too much stress upon themselves. Tell the second type of muscles that they can hand over some of their stress, and tell the entire muscular system that some muscles will take up more stress and others less, and that the whole procedure will be experienced as a relief.

Muscular tension can be relieved by suggesting to the body that it should follow an internal model of muscular stress distribution and transfer tension from the muscles which have been overloaded to date to those which have been underloaded.

Work on the rigging

T: **Lumbago, muscular tension, snoring, torticollis**
R: **The dock workers within the muscular system**
M: **You know how to redistribute tension. Do your job and do it well!**

After a sailing ship has weathered a storm, it sails into a dock so that all the rigging can be tuned up. The cordage is loosened and tightened and then loosened again and tightened again, over and over again until everything is just right. Please tell the workers that they're doing a great job!

It goes without saying that greetings can also be integrated into metaphors or parables, allowing inner persons within the body to be addressed in metaphorical form as individuals who should be supported in their work.

Pain

"Pain is optional,"[29] and it can often be reduced using relatively simple methods. Astonishingly enough, most adults are able and willing to teach pre-schoolers simple rituals to relieve the pain of a scuffed knee or other minor injuries, but fail to connect the dots and apply similar rituals when they experience pain themselves. Even the few adults who have developed pain reduction techniques which they use during dental treatment or similar tests of endurance tend not to talk about it with others, and do not transfer these techniques to other areas of their lives.

Greetings are an excellent way of reducing and relieving pain, since the job of bringing about helpful changes is entrusted not to the thinking mind, but to unconscious persons within the body who are far better suited to this task.

In my opinion, there is no value in distinguishing between "psychosomatic" and "purely somatic" pain, or in concluding on this basis that greetings can only help with pain of the first type. In my experience, therapeutic work with clients who suffer from pain-related symptoms is easier if there are fewer links between the pain experienced in the body and internal or external conflicts, and more complex if the stressful situations that might be associated with the pain are diverse in nature, recent or threatening; the intensity of the pain experience depends on psychological factors even in the case of what appears to be "purely somatic" pain.

Headache in the waiting room

T: **Pain**

R: **Headache**

M: **You're welcome, but you're not welcome here. I will take notice of you, but not now – later.**

> Send a greeting to your headache, and tell it that it is welcome to stay for a while if it likes, but it should go and wait in the big toe on your right foot until you are ready. Don't forget to say thank you![30]

Headaches are unpopular despite their useful role in drawing the sufferer's attention to certain physical or emotional needs which are not being met. The greeting, the expression of gratitude and the permission to remain break down the sufferer's defences, and at the same time probably also reduce the stress which caused or worsened the headache. The message expressed in the greeting is that the headache can be moved to a location in the body where it is less in the way, and the encounter with pain can be put off to some point in the future. The symptom is encouraged to adopt a passive attitude ("wait"), which suggests that the client should play a more creative role in return. In interventions which consist of a series of whimsical suggestions, each new suggestion distracts the client from any temptation to discuss or critically examine the one before, ensuring that the content of the message is implemented yet more effectively.

Distorted time

T: **Pain (pulsating)**
R: **The body**
M: **You can accelerate your subjective experience of time during periods of suffering and decelerate it during periods without suffering, so that you have a more pleasant time of it in general.**

> Sometimes hours pass in the blink of an eye, and minutes stretch out into an eternity. Send a greeting to your body, and ask it to experience time as accelerated whenever it feels the pulsating pain, and to experience time as decelerated during the periods in between, more and more effectively each time. Has anything changed?

The procedure is based on an intervention by Milton Erickson.[31]

During an experiment I carried out on myself, a pulsating pain I had experienced in my foot for months disappeared in a matter of seconds. Building on this experiment, I began to consider how the phenomenon of time distortion could be used on a flexible basis to influence the frequency, duration and intensity of the symptoms experienced by clients.

The good intention returns

T: **Anxiety, pain, worry, anaesthesia**
R: **The person inside you who knows what pain feels like**
M: **If you take a personified version of the pain out of you, and only allow its good intentions to return, the way your body feels will change.**

Paint a picture in your mind of the person inside you who knows what pain feels like, and imagine that this person is leaving your body, invisibly standing up and walking over to the door, leaving you sitting there – is that a pleasant thing to imagine, or would you rather have the person back? Perhaps we could ask that person to stay over there and only to allow the good intentions behind the pain to return to you – how would that feel?

I developed the intervention when dealing with a client suffering from osteoarthrosis of the shoulder. Several attempts to anaesthetise his pain at a psychological level failed, until I allowed the good intentions behind the symptoms, "whatever they might be," to return to him without the experience of pain. When I asked the client what the good intentions of the symptoms had been, he said, "the pain wanted to prevent me from overstraining my shoulder." A little while later, when working with a client who was suffering from the same symptoms, I introduced this distinction at the very start of the course of therapy, with the same positive outcome. Interventions of this kind – sending a personified version of the stress out of the client's body, and only allowing the good intentions to return – have also proven successful for anxiety disorders and other problems which tend to be psychological in nature.

Hearing

The interventions in this section are designed for use with clients suffering from tinnitus and hearing loss. Tinnitus presents in a huge variety of ways, and so it is important for any treatment plan to be just as unique as the symptoms being treated. It is generally the case that clients suffering from tinnitus were subject to high levels of stress in their lives at the time when the symptoms first occurred. Treatment has a higher chance of success if the client can be taught to respond relatively calmly and serenely to stress triggers of this kind and to memories of their past stressful experiences.

Ear cleaning

T: **Cold, hearing loss, hearing impairment, thrombosis, tinnitus**
R: **The body**
M: **You can reduce your hearing loss using a secret method which is known only to your body, and which cannot be explained by rational logic or research findings.**

I'm afraid that your ear canals are clogged up with gunk, all the way through to your brain. Have you ever come across the rodents known as bristly mice? Tell your body that it should send some bristly mice backwards through your ear canals – through the wide ones for the low tones and the narrow ones for the high tones – making sure that they are tilted slightly to the side so that the mice's spiky bristles can clean out all the gunk in there, and they can then wipe off the small bits of dust with their whiskers. When the mice have finished their job, your body can then rinse your ear canals out using plenty of bodily fluid. Check and see what they did – is everything OK now, or do we need wire-haired mice?

The greeting can be used in connection with various types of hearing impairment and tinnitus, and often leads to a subjective improvement in symptoms (and frequently one which can be measured using psychoacoustic methods). The greeting played a central role in a one-hour treatment session which led to the full remission of the hearing loss and tinnitus symptoms which a seminar participant had been experiencing for several months.[32]

Communication among the bristly mice

T: **Hearing loss, hearing impairment, tinnitus**
R: **Bristly mice**
M: **I can help you to help me! The things which previously bothered me have a purpose and form part of my treatment.**

Bristly mice have to be good communicators so that they don't bump into each other in all those dark passageways. They need to get better and better at recognising tiny differences in high tones and low tones, in the rustling of their bristles on the walls and in the volume of the noises. You can help them by paying attention and becoming skilled yourself at accurately recognising the tiny differences between pitches, volumes and silences.

Tinnitus sufferers who actively concentrate on differences in pitch and volume may find that the tinnitus noises and accompanying hearing impairment are reduced or eliminated, and so it is often helpful to teach them (either openly or covertly) the skills needed to hear these differences. Tinnitus noises which are interpreted as a useful form of communication become less threatening, which in turn lessens the compulsive thoughts that tend to perpetuate these noises ("Can I still hear them? Can I still hear them?"). Clients report an increasing tendency to "forget" that the noises are there as a result.

Say hello to your ear

T: **Tinnitus**
R: **The ear**
M: **I tolerate the things I cannot forbid. I tolerate the things I forbid. Silence and peace are two different things. Feel free to bleep away quietly; the seemingly impossible is possible.**

I'd like to start by asking you to pass on the following message to your ear: "You can beep away quietly, but leave me in peace!"

Instead of attempting to fight tinnitus and potentially stabilising it in the process, a therapeutic double bind is used; the noise is both welcomed and asked to be quiet. It is so difficult to understand what this might mean that it is hard to agree to the proposal but also hard to object to it, and so once the conscious mind has tried and failed to assess the significance of the double message in the greeting, the unconscious mind will look for a way in which the greeting might be implemented. The two different sides of the ambivalence which is presumed to be at the heart of the problem are given their due; it is acknowledged that the noise is associated with good intentions of some kind, or in other words that it has a reason to exist, but also that it is bothering the sufferer and needs to be put in its place. The double bind between the two halves of the sentence is foreshadowed in the first half; "beep away quietly" is a contradiction, at least in terms of meaning. "You can" also has a double meaning: either "you may" or "you are able."

The five scientific observers

T: **Tinnitus**

R: **The controlling one, the annoyed one, the one with objections, the perfectionist and the one who wants to drown something out (five recipients with five tasks)**

M: **Everyone who contributes to the problem is given a new place to stand and assigned a new task. The work carried out will deliver a result which can be documented and which is scientifically recognised.**

I'd like to call on some scientific observers to help us with our task – experts who document the outcome rather than influencing it. Imagine that up until now there has been someone inside you who controlled whether the noise was still there, and put him over there. There was also someone else who used to get annoyed by the noise, so we'll imagine that the controlling one puts him somewhere nearby. Then there was someone who had objections and doubted whether it would all work, and so the annoyed one put him right there. The one with objections puts the perfectionist – the one inside you who would accept nothing less than a complete and immediate miracle – over there. Finally, the perfectionist puts the one inside you who wants to drown out emotional pain of some kind over there, and asks him to anaesthetise the pain using a different method in future. Look at the five of them over there – the controlling one, the annoyed one, the one with objections, the perfectionist and the one who wants to drown something out. Look inside yourself to see what has changed now that they are all over there instead of inside you, and then we can get started.

To begin with, all of the inner persons who play a role in the acoustic phenomenon are spatially dissociated and given different tasks. Only then does work on the tinnitus begin, in a trance of confusion which makes it difficult for them to control the noise.

Fine-tune your hearing

T: **Tinnitus**
R: **The auditory cortex**
M: **Learn to perceive smaller differences in frequencies and volumes in the vicinity of the tinnitus noises and the adjacent hearing loss.**

There are certain frequency ranges where you can't hear things very well, and so your hearing turns up the perceived volume – and it's in the zones which are immediately next to these ranges that tinnitus occurs. In a landscape of vertiginous drops, where you can sometimes hear everything which is a tenth of a semitone lower and almost nothing which is a tenth of a semitone higher, your brain turns up the volume for the frequency range in which you have trouble hearing, and accidently does the same for the adjacent range in which you can hear perfectly well. Tell the auditory cortex in your brain that it should regulate the frequencies and volumes in this range more accurately, so that it is better at distinguishing differences in the hearing it generates than in the sounds it generates.

The brain can learn to perceive differences in volume and pitch (passive reception) just as easily as it can generate different volumes and pitches (active production). The purpose of the greeting is to tell the unconscious mind not to confuse frequency ranges in which the hearing is impaired with adjacent frequency ranges (in which there is no impairment of hearing) when turning up the volume to overcome the impairment. When the intensity of noise in the tinnitus frequency ranges is reduced, the level of hearing impairment in the adjacent frequency ranges is also automatically reduced; learning how to distinguish more accurately between volumes and pitches improves the ability to hear silence just as much as the ability to hear noise.

Loud and quiet, high and low

T: **Tinnitus**
R: **The ear**
M: **You are getting better and better at perceiving differences in pitch and volume. The more you succeed in doing so, the quieter the noises become.**

> Please tell your ear that it should listen more and more carefully to my voice as I speak, without being prompted to do so, and try to get better and better at perceiving the differences in pitch and volume. After our session today ends, it should continue to do the same thing, but with other sounds and noises. The more skilled it becomes at perceiving these differences, the fewer phantom noises it will experience.

The greeting helps to regulate hearing problems in the frequency range adjacent to the tinnitus noises and simultaneously reduces these noises.

Turn it around to make a sound!

T: **Tinnitus**
R: **The auditory centre**
M: **The noise is always there, and the brain is responsible for creating silence. The soundproof door is open. Close it!**

> Strictly speaking, it's the other way around; your brain constantly has to deal with absolute pandemonium on all of the different frequencies, and it uses soundproof doors to create silence. Whenever you hear a sound, your brain has opened and closed one of these soundproof doors and interrupted the silence. Tell your auditory centre that one of the doors is ajar or not quite soundproof, and that it needs to be closed properly – thank you!

The intervention switches the client's focus from listening for noises to listening for silence.

Retraining the bodyguard

T: **Tinnitus**
R: **The ear**
M: **The tinnitus is welcome to return when the stressful situation which first triggered it also returns. Until then, it should stay away.**

> You first experienced tinnitus symptoms during a period when you were going through a stressful situation. Perhaps this situation was more stressful for you than others might think, because it reminded you of a time way back in your past when you experienced something similar, and this multiplied the stress. Tell your ear that if these events are repeated again – the events you've been reminded of by the recent situation, and which have triggered the noises in your ear – it is welcome to raise the alarm. Until then, it can remain at ease.

The tinnitus is framed as an alarm signal in response to stressful situations which subliminally remind the client of earlier and more serious stresses, i.e. essentially as a response to traumatic triggers. The client is invited to consider the possibility that the tinnitus has continued to exist even though the original context has been forgotten because it has some kind of intrinsic value. The suggestion is then put forwards that a distinction should be made firstly between the alarm signal and the current stressful situation, and secondly between the current stressful situation and the original events. No attempt is made to fight the tinnitus; instead, it is proposed that it should continue in its current role, but only raise the alarm if the stressful situation which first triggered it returns.

Fire detector

T: **Tinnitus**
R: **The ear**
M: **We can agree on the value of the sound as an alarm signal, but alarms are only effective if they are turned off once the danger has passed.**

> Send a greeting to your ear, and tell it that the fire has been extinguished and the fire detector can be turned off. But don't forget that if a fire alarm goes off in a large building, it doesn't get turned off immediately by the first person who comes along; an expert is called in who inspects all the fire detectors once business is over for the day, carries out any maintenance operations required and reconfigures them.

Although it is hard to deny the logic underlying this metaphor, only a few lucky clients will report back that the noise was switched off immediately, since the inner person within the body responsible for switching off the noise is also responsible for switching it on. Reference is therefore made to the fact that the ear or another inner entity should call in an expert who will handle the problem more professionally than the client "once business is over for the day," i.e. when he or she is either asleep or relaxed and distracted.

Other somatic issues

The interventions outlined in this section can be used to treat a variety of disorders, and also serve as a basis for developing greeting-style interventions for use in contexts not mentioned in this book.

Carpal tunnel syndrome

T: **Carpal tunnel syndrome**
R: **The body**
M: **You can adjust the mobility of your tendons.**

Tendons have a sheath, and they move around in this sheath just like a bicycle brake cable moves around in its tubing. Send a greeting to your body, and tell it to make the cable thinner and the tubing wider, and to put a tiny drop of oil on the brake cable – thank you! Now enjoy moving your fingers!

This intervention was first used during a conversation with a woman who was suffering from thumb mobility problems, and who was not happy with her GP's recommendation to put up with it because it was simply part of ageing. The greeting led to a significant improvement within a matter of seconds, and the symptoms disappeared entirely after the use of several follow-up greetings over the next few days and weeks.

The right/left conference

T: **Multiple sclerosis, stroke**
R: **The right-hand and left-hand sides of the body, in relation to each other**
M: **The mobile half of the body can teach the paralysed half how to move.**

How does the right half of your body manage to do such a good job of moving? The right-hand and left-hand sides of your body have sent teams of representatives to a right/left conference, where they meet in working groups and the right-siders show the left-siders how movement works. The team representing the right leg shows the team representing the left leg how to move the correct muscles, and the team for the right-hand side of the face gives the team for the left-hand side of the face an introduction to the art of movement. In the evening they all go out dancing together. What do the left-siders learn from the right-siders, and what teaching methods do the right-siders use so that the left-siders can learn as effectively as possible?

The purpose of the greeting is to enhance communication between parts of the body that are working well and those that are not working so well, and to restore the bodily functions on the left-hand side of the body through a process of copying those on the right-hand side.

Advanced personal hygiene

T: **Thrombosis, arteriosclerosis**
R: **Someone in your brain**
M: **Clean your veins regularly and with particular care.**

How often do you clean your teeth? There is someone in your brain who knows how to use a toothbrush, regardless of whether the task at hand involves cleaning teeth or a rusty old lock or a clock mechanism. Send a greeting to this someone, and tell him or her that he or she should give your veins and the valves in your veins a good polish whenever you clean your teeth.

This intervention was developed during a conversation with an acquaintance, who told me something that her GP had said: apparently the blood looks for alternative routes after a venous thrombosis, and the valves in the veins do not usually regain their full range of functioning. Since I was recovering from a deep vein thrombosis myself at the time, I experimented by imagining to myself the cleaning procedure described here on a daily basis, in particular at the locations where I felt a pinching or pressing sensation. It is impossible to prove whether the intervention had any effect on the healing process, but my phlebologist could find no residual symptoms when I returned for a check-up six months later.

Couples and family therapy

Greetings can be used in couples and family therapy just as effectively as in individual therapy. The recipient of the greeting can be an entity within one of the partners ("Please send a greeting to your mind, Ms X"), an entity in each of the two partners ("Please send greetings to your minds, Ms X and Mr X") or the couple as a single unit ("Please send a greeting to the couple that you once were" or ". . . that you will be in future" or ". . . that you could be, and that is happier than you knew was possible").

In exceptional cases where the therapist is working with only one of the partners in a couple, the other partner can be externalised as "the image of your partner in your head," and also function as the recipient of greetings in this form. One way of doing this is outlined in the greeting "The couple in his head." A similar procedure can be used to create mental representations of other family and team members in the mind of the client who is present with the therapist.

Angels and other invisible friends can also be assigned the role of bearers of greetings when working with families and children; one such approach is described in the greeting "Heavenly homework helper."

The unhappy couple out there

T: **Relationships**
R: **The unhappy couple outside the partners who are physically present**
M: **The experience of being unhappy does not need to be in the same location as the couple that is physically present. Even if the physically present couple is no longer suffering, we can consider the possibility of being an unhappy couple.**

Imagine that the couple that can't help arguing with each other every day stands up, leaves both of your bodies invisibly, and sits down over there, just to the left of you. . . . Now you two look a lot more relaxed, but the opposite is true for those two over there! The pair of you don't really need much more in the way of therapy, but the other couple certainly do. I'd like to send a message to the couple over there; we're just going to have a little chat over here for a while, and then we'll deal with them.

When the unhappy couple is dissociated from the couple that is physically present, the latter can experience – typically with some astonishment – their partnership independently of the unhappiness with which it is usually associated. In order to distract the partners from the idea that the stress must necessarily return, the invisible unhappy couple is also offered therapy, so that even if it later finds its way back into the identity of the physically present couple, it will have been transformed from an unhappy into a relatively happy couple.

Your suffering as a bodyguard

T: **Trauma, relationships**
R: **The person within you who experienced something similar as a child**
M: **Make sure that the earlier event never happens again.**

> I understand that you have gone through some tough times together. If there happens to be someone inside you, Ms N, who experienced something similar a long time ago, perhaps during childhood, I'd like to ask this person to watch over you like a bodyguard and make sure that the terrible thing which happened so long ago never happens again.

Recognising the value behind traumatic triggers, differentiating them from the self and narrowing down their purpose to preventing the original events from occurring again ensures that situations which are only similar (rather than identical) to the original traumatic events need no longer be interpreted as alarming or retraumatising.

Two good bodyguards

T: **Trauma, relationships**
R: **The persons inside both of you who experienced something similar as a child**
M: **You can help your host bodies by only raising the alarm when the things which are happening right now are exactly the same as they were back then.**

> And if there happens to be someone inside you, Mr N, who experienced something similar a long time ago, perhaps during childhood,

I'd also like to ask this person to watch over you like a bodyguard. Both of your bodyguards are doing a great job, and they should keep up the good work. In order to make life easier for themselves, they should only raise the alarm when the things which are happening right now are exactly the same as they were back then.

This intervention follows the same approach as "Retraining the bodyguard" from the section on hearing, and simply transfers it to two partners and their interactions.

The couple in your head

T: **Relationships**
R: **The couple in your head**
M: **If the story of your relationship which you tell yourself in your head has a happy ending, the same might happen in real life.**

In your head you have an image of your husband, of yourself and of your relationship. It's time for the couple in your head to get outside for once – send them off on a journey through a world of infinite opportunities for building a healthy relationship, and let them grow alongside one another for 100 years on earth and 100 years in heaven. Do you think they might treat each other very differently when they come back?

The intervention is similar to "Journey to heaven" in the section on trauma; it differs only in that two people are sent on the journey together in this case.

The couple in his head

T: **Relationship**
R: **The couple in your head**
M: **The altered couple in your head and the unaltered couple in his head will gradually grow to resemble each other. Make sure that the couple in your head is much better at enforcing their way of doing things than the couple in his head could ever be.**

Your husband is not here today, but he too has an image of himself, of you and of your relationship in his head. The images in your head and in his head will tend to align themselves automatically over time. If the couple in your head, who have journeyed through heaven and earth for 200 years, are ready to love each other and act more kindly to each other than the couple in his head, this process of automatic alignment might get tricky. Send a greeting to the couple in your head, and tell them that they should not be influenced by the couple in his head, which has not been on the same journey. They need to be patient until the couple in his head has come around to this new and more agreeable way of doing things.

Therapy which involves a couple "in the client's head" has a better chance of lasting success if the therapist states that the two couples typically meet in the middle, so that 50% of the therapeutic effect is retained, but that the mind is capable of ensuring that the altered couple is better at enforcing its way of doing things than the unaltered.

Heavenly homework helper

T: **School, homework**
R: **You, via an angel**
M: **It is not up to us as parents to nag you about doing your homework – invisible third parties can do it wisely, lovingly and discreetly.**

Later I will send you an angel who will remind you to do your homework.

The greeting was developed by a seminar participant who regularly assigned a heavenly messenger the conflict-ridden task of reminding his family members to do their homework.

Notes

1 Cf. Zeig 1985, 50, 64, 66, 73, 95 et passim for further details of Milton Erickson's approach.
2 Hammel 2014, 42–50, 65–85, Hammel 2019b, 26. For further details of the therapeutic use of fragmentation by Erickson, cf. Short & Weinspach 2007, 108–131.

3 Hammel 2014, 290.
4 Ibid.
5 Ibid.
6 Hammel 2016a, 69.
7 Ibid., 87.
8 Cf. Hammel 2014, 192.
9 Hammel 2011, 218–223, Short & Weinspach 2007, 250–263, Erickson, Rossi & Rossi, 1976, 62–76. Erickson & Rossi 1981, 70, 88, 157, 172.
10 Based on Hammel 2014, 192–193.
11 Ibid.
12 Ibid., 195.
13 See the sections on depression and sleep.
14 Hammel 2014, 196.
15 I developed this intervention in collaboration with a client who told me what I should do with his residual psychosis following a psychotic episode.
16 Cf. Hammel 2019a, 83–84.
17 Cf. Hammel 2009, 180 f. To read more about the idea of achieving a balance between giving and taking, cf. Weber 1997, 22–39.
18 Hammel 2014, 291.
19 Ibid.
20 Another method of reconditioning sleep behaviours associated with nightmares can be found in Hammel 2019a, 83–84.
21 A test reader of the manuscript of this book sent me the following message: "I tried out the greeting with the snoring angel immediately. My husband is extremely grateful to you."
22 A more detailed description of the procedure can be found in Hammel 2016a, 84.
23 Cf. Hammel 2014, 30.
24 Ibid., 290–291.
25 Hammel 2016a, 56.
26 Based on numerous medical cases, Salomon Sellam describes dissociated traumatic experiences ("psy-choc émotionel déstabilisant") as common triggers of allergies: "Dans la quasi-totalité des histoires d'allergie il existe un . . . episode [destabilisant à l'origine du déclenchement des symptomes] plus ou moins occulté aujourd'hui" (Sellam 2005, 37). He states that the allergen is always directly associated with a previous hazardous situation which has been blocked out, and serves as a warning of a different hazard which is known in principle but has been dissociated: "L'allergéne . . . est toujours accolé à une situation de danger précédement ressenti comme telle. . . . L'allergéne n'est qu'un simple avertisseur de l'imminence d'un danger dèjà connu, mais occulté." The observation that mourning, trauma and severe inner conflicts can trigger allergies is also pointed out by Unterberger, Wilcke & Witt, 23–28, who give further case examples.
27 Hammel 2012, 51.
28 Cf. "Retraining the bodyguard" in the section on hearing, for example.
29 "Pain is optional" stated Dan Kohen, when presenting the outcomes of a long-term study on the effectiveness of hypnotherapy in children and young people suffering from migraines, at the 2009 Children's Conference in Heidelberg.
30 Hammel 2014, 291.
31 O'Hanlon & Hexum 1990, 65–66. Cf. Hammel 2019a, 59–60.

32 Hypnotherapeutic training seminar in Kaiserslautern in November 2016. When working with the seminar participant in question, we discussed not only bristly mice but also the emotionally stressful situation which the participant was currently facing and which she had experienced during a previous episode of hearing loss three years ago, as well as once during childhood.

List of greetings

Bibliography

Alman, B., & Lambrou, P. (1999). *Self-Hypnosis: The Complete Guide to Better Health and Self-Change*. London, New York: Routledge.

Bandler, R., & Grinder, J. (1991). *Trance-Formations: Neuro-Linguistic Programming and the Structure of Hypnosis*. Boulder, CO: Real People.

Beebe, B., Jaffe, J., Lachmann, F., Feldstein, S., Crown, C., & Jasnow, M. (2002). Koordination von Sprachrhythmus und Bindung: Systemtheoretische Modelle, in: Brisch, K. H., Grossmann, K. E., & Köhler, L. (eds.): *Bindung und seelische Entwicklungswege*. Stuttgart: Klett-Cotta, 47–87.

Erickson, M., & Rossi, E. (1979). *Hypnotherapy: An Exploratory Casebook*. New York: Irvington.

Erickson, M., & Rossi, E. (1981). *Experiencing Hypnosis: Therapeutic Approaches to Altered States by Milton H. Erickson*. New York: Irvington.

Erickson, M., Rossi, E., & Rossi, S. (1976). *Hypnotic Realities: The Introduction of Clinical Hypnosis and Forms of Indirect Suggestion*. New York: Irvington.

Gordon, D., & Meyers-Anderson, M. (2018). *Phoenix: Therapeutic Patterns of Milton H. Erickson*. Tucson: David Gordon.

Haley, J. (1993). *Uncommon Therapy: The Psychiatric Techniques of Milton H. Erickson, M.D.* New York: Norton.

Haley, J. (2011). *Ordeal-Therapy: Unusual Ways to Change Behavior*. Bancyfelin: Crown House.

Hammel, S. (2009). Tinnitustherapie durch Hypnose: Der Heidelberger Pilotversuch. *Musica Sacra*, 04/09, 223–226.

Hammel, S. (2010). Von Möwenfelsen und Felsenbirnen: Aufbruchsgeschichten für Kinder und Jugendliche. *Familiendynamik*, 2, 136–143.

Hammel, S. (2011). *Handbuch der therapeutischen Utilisation: Vom Nutzen des Unnützen in Psychotherapie, Kinder- und Familientherapie, Heilkunde und Beratung*. Stuttgart: Klett-Cotta.

Hammel, S. (2012a). Metapher, in: Kleve, H., & Wirth, J. (eds.): *Lexikon des systemischen Arbeitens: Grundbegriffe der Systemischen Praxis, Methodik und Theorie*. Heidelberg: Carl Auer, 264–267.

Hammel, S. (2012b). Utilisation, in: Kleve, H., & Wirth, J. (eds.): *Lexikon des systemischen Arbeitens. Grundbegriffe der Systemischen Praxis, Methodik und Theorie*. Heidelberg: Carl Auer, 441–444.

Hammel, S. (2012c). *The Blade of Grass in the Desert: Storytelling: Forgotten Medicine for Healing the Soul. A Story of 100 Stories for Counseling and Therapy.* Nierstein: impress.

Hammel, S. (2014). *Therapie zwischen den Zeilen: Das ungesagt Gesagte in Beratung, Therapie und Heilkunde.* Stuttgart: Klett-Cotta.

Hammel, S. (2016a). *Alles neu gerahmt! Psychische Symptome in ungewöhnlicher Perspektive.* München: Ernst Reinhardt.

Hammel, S. (2016b). *Loslassen und leben: Befreiende Geschichten.* Nierstein: impress.

Hammel, S. (2018). *The Island of Love: A Game for Couple Therapy.* Kaiserslautern: HSB.

Hammel, S. (2019a). *Handbook of Therapeutic Storytelling: Stories and Metaphors in Psychotherapy, Child and Family Therapy, Medical Treatment, Coaching and Supervision.* London, New York: Routledge.

Hammel, S. (2019b). *Lebensmöglichkeiten entdecken: Veränderungen durch Therapeutisches Modellieren.* Stuttgart: Klett-Cotta.

Hammel, S. (2019c). *Therapeutic Storytelling and Therapeutic Modeling in Couple Therapy: DVD-Documentation of a Single Session on a 1.5 hr Congress Workshop.* Kaiserslautern: HSB.

Hammel, S. (2019d). *The Art of Therapeutic Storytelling: Audio Recording of an Introductory Workshop (Glasgow 2018).* Kaiserslautern: HSB.

Hammel, S., Hürzeler, A., Lamprecht, K., & Niedermann, M. (2015). *Wie das Krokodil zum Fliegen kam: 120 Geschichten, die das Leben verändern.* München: Ernst Reinhardt.

Hammel, S., Hürzeler, A., Lamprecht, K., & Niedermann, M. (2018). *Wie der Bär zum Fliegen kam: 120 Geschichten für einen gesunden Körper.* München: Ernst Reinhardt.

Hammond, D. (ed.) (1990). *Handbook of Therapeutic Suggestions and Metaphors.* New York: Norton.

Hesse, P. U. (2003). *Teilearbeit: Konzepte von Multiplizität in ausgewählten Bereichen moderner Psychotherapie.* Heidelberg: Carl Auer.

Loriedo, C., & Vella, G. (2011). *Paradox and the Family System.* London, New York: Routledge.

Meiss, O. (2016). *Hypnosystemische Therapie bei Depression und Burnout.* Heidelberg: Carl Auer.

O'Hanlon, H., & Hexum, A. (1990). *An Uncommon Casebook: The Complete Clinical Work of Milton H. Erickson, M.D.* New York: Norton.

Olness, K., & Kohen, D. (2011). *Hypnosis and Hypnotherapy with Children.* London, New York: Routledge.

Prior, M. (2007). *Beratung und Therapie optimal vorbereiten: Informationen und Interventionen vor dem ersten Gespräch.* Heidelberg: Carl Auer.

Prior, M. (2017). *MiniMax Interventions: 15 Simple Therapeutic Interventions That Have Maximum Impact.* Bancyfelin: Crown House.

Rosen, S. (ed.) (1982). *My Voice Will Go with You: Teaching Tales of Milton H. Erickson.* New York: Norton.

Rossi, E. (ed.) (2008–10). *Collected Works of Milton H. Erickson* (6 Volumes). Phoenix: Milton H. Erickson Foundation Press.

Schmidt, G. (2014). *Einführung in die hypnosystemische Therapie und Beratung.* Heidelberg: Carl Auer.

Schneider, P. (2009). Musik, von Engeln vorgesungen: Entstehung und Ursachen von Tinnitus und Geräuschempfindlichkeit bei Kirchenmusikern, Chorleitern, Bläsern und Sängern. Musica Sacra, 04/09, 220–222.

Schneider, P., Andermann, M., Wengenroth, M., Goebel, R., Flor, H., Rupp, A., & Diesch, E. (2009). Reduced Volume of Heschl's Gyrus in Tinnitus. *Neuroimage,* 45, 927–939.

Schulz von Thun, F., & Stegemann, W. (eds.) (2004). *Das innere Team in Aktion: Praktische Arbeit mit dem Modell.* Reinbek: Rowohlt.

Schwartz, R. (1995). *Internal Family Systems Therapy.* New York, London: Guilford.

Sellam, S. (2005). *Les allergies. C'est plus simple qu'on le pense.* Bérangel: Saint André de Sangonis.

Short, D., & Weinspach, C. (2007). *Hoffnung und Resilenz: therapeutische Strategien von Milton Erickson.* Heidelberg: Carl Auer.

Unterberger, G., Wilcke, I., & Witt, K. (2014). *Allergien mental behandeln: Damit Geist und Körper wieder angemessen reagieren können – Modelle und Strategien angewandter Psychoneuroimmunologie.* Bargteheide: Psymed.

Watzlawick, P. (1976). *How Real Is Real? Confusion, Disinformation, Communication.* New York: Random House.

Watzlawick, P., Jackson, D., & Beavin Bavelas, J. (1976). *Pragmatics of Human Communication: A Study of Interactional Patterns, Pathologies and Paradoxes.* New York: Norton.

Weber, G. (ed.) (1997). *Zweierlei Glück. Die systemische Psychotherapie Bert Hellingers.* Heidelberg: Carl Auer.

Zeig, J. K. (1985). *Experiencing Erickson. An Introduction to the Man and his Work.* New York: Brunner, Mazel.

Zeig, J. K. (ed.) (1999). *A Teaching Seminar with Milton H. Erickson.* London, New York: Routledge.

Index